Food, Fitness, and Fulfillment

A Fitness book by Lester Albright

Table of Contents

Chapter 1.) Introduction

Chapter 2.) Motivation

Chapter 3.) Weekly Gym Workout Plan

Chapter 4.) Five-day Diet Plan

Chapter 5.) Reducing Body Fat

Chapter 6.) Breathing Techniques

Chapter 7.) Recommendation of Protein Intake

Chapter 8.) Recommended Juice Combinations for Health

Chapter 9.) Stress Reduction

Chapter 10) Warm-up Routine

Chapter 11.) Weekly Home Workout Plan

Chapter 12.) Obesity Amongst Youth

Chapter 13.) Acknowledgments

Chapter 1

Introduction

This book is written for the experienced fitness buff as well as the inexperienced trainee. In it there are useful techniques that may, if applied rigorously, offer lifetime benefits. It is a guideline for complete and total wellness incorporating physical training and nutrition. Depending on your level of experience, the recommendations can be adjusted during your sessions. If you are seeking to develop more muscle mass, it is essential to utilize reps of 8-10 and heavier, but controlled, weight so that your form and technique is correct. By utilizing controlled weight you will be able to isolate the targeted muscle that is considered the "primary" muscle. You will find that some of these routines focus on exercises where two muscle groups complement one another. For example, if you were to do a chest routine the chest would be the primary muscle and the triceps would become the secondary muscle affected because the range of motion used in pushing off from the chest isolates the triceps during extension.

Dieting can be an important aspect of fitness however overall nutrition management must be used in conjunction with exercise to increase the opportunity for success in reaching your personal goals. Included in this book is a five-day workout regimen along with a five-day diet plan. As stated earlier, these methods can be used for as long as you chose to train and can have lifetime benefits. Calisthenics are also recommended as part of a good fitness regimen for the strength endurance that supports lifting or pushing ones own natural body weight and can also be used in preparation for weight training.

Although these methods are recommendations that can lead to great results in training and fitness it is highly suggested that a physician is consulted when considering and before beginning any physical exercise, training, or dieting. Consideration must be given to any medical conditions or physical restrictions that may apply. The author does not guarantee results for all individuals and is not liable for results as the information offered are suggestions alone. The nutritional advice recommended in this book has not been approved by the FDA or any physician. Any suggestions given are based on personal research as well as experience.

I wish you Blessings and great success with your training. I pray you reach your desired goal and reap the benefits of maintaining positive health consciousness. When we view fitness as part of a contribution to overall good health and not just for its physical benefits it is an expression of our appreciation for the gift of life that God has given each one of us. Thank you for considering this book sincerely the athuor.

Chapter 2

Motivation

There are many people who do not involve themselves in fitness training for several reasons. Those reasons may vary and they all have some validity. Lack of energy, busy schedules, finances, and lack of knowledge about fitness are just a few. However, these reasons can also be excuses and no excuse is good enough when it comes to personal health. We must be mindful of the importance of good health and how it applies to us.

Health is not something that we can afford to take for granted nor can we afford to neglect for it affects every aspect of our lives. Great health is one of the most precious gifts God has given us. With it the benefits are great for living active and fulfilling lives. If you seek to improve your life and its effectiveness, fitness and diet are two key areas of focus to which it can be achieved. Once an individual begins a serious fitness regimen healthy diet and nutrition will follow. In turn, resulting from the tenacity of the individual in improving those areas other undesirable habits or patterns of living are overcome.

As the human body ages bone and joints wear thus becoming more susceptible to injury. Organs have been subjected to the same fact. Proper nutrition and exercise can decrease the occurrences of illness and injury and promote longevity.

Benjamin Franklin stated, "An ounce of prevention is worth a pound of cure". I am, in essence, saying the same thing. If we are motivated to engage in some form of fitness and have good eating habits there will be less chance of virus causing bacteria invading our bodies. Many health issues affecting our society today can be managed and controlled if some time in our busy schedules is given to the things I am suggesting. Financially, the cost of medical visits and hospitalizations could be reduced to routine check-ups with a physician.

Cardiovascular training can aid in maintaining blood pressure and weight loss. It also stimulates blood flow to the heart and arteries. Strength and conditioning training creates stronger, healthier, bones and joints. Complimenting the two with a good diet plan will not only improve how you feel but how you look also. Because people are generally encouraged more by what is seen as opposed to what is said, imagine how many family, friends, and loved ones that could be encouraged to do the same by your results. Even those individuals that do not verbalize it will be inspired by your overall better, happier appearance and mood.

So I challenge you today to live a better, healthier, more enjoyable life for you, your family, friends, and loved ones. The knowledge you will receive in this book is yours for life. Feel free to pass it on to those you wish great health!

Chapter 3

Weekly Gym Workout Plan

Day One (1) Chest and Triceps:

The chest routine will begin with a basic flat bench with the straight bar. Utilizing only the bar you can warm up being sure to focus on form and technique. After doing so, depending on the amount of weight you are conditioned to lifting you can set your bar and begin.

If you are a beginner you're presently in strength and conditioning phase. If the goal is to build more muscle mass I recommend 8-10 reps using heavy weight as sufficient, and reps of 12-15 with less weight if you desire more toning or sculpting muscle. This can be repeated for a minimum of three sets. There are three exercises that are designed for developing the upper (clavicular head) and lower (sternal head) chest. The incline, flat, and decline, benches. Together these exercises will give you a total straight bar routine. Another option is a dumbbell workout. The **dumbbell workout** focuses on more shape and can be done in flat, incline, and decline positions.

The **pec machine** is another great exercise for the chest. When conducting this exercise be sure to contract the pectoral muscles when the hands are conjoined and stretch the muscles when cables are released. This routine can be repeated for a minimum of three sets with reps of 12-15 depending on individual goals. The next exercise for day one will be for triceps.

First, there is the **cable pull down** exercise using the curl bar, straight bar, or rope cables. Starting with your elbows at your sides, and arms raised at a 45-degree angle, pull cables in downward position. Once in this position, contract the tricep portion of the arm. Keep arms in this position for approximately one second to allow the blood to settle in the targeted muscle. Raise arms back to start position and repeat motion for a minimum of three sets. Reps will vary based on desired goal.

Skull crushes can be done with the curl bar. While lying down on the weight bench with bar held above the chest (hands outward and elbows locked) slowly lower the bar, using only the forearm and being sure that the elbows remain pointed in an upright position. Once the bar is slightly above the forehead return to your starting position. Repeat rotation for a minimum of three sets. Again, reps will vary based on desired goal. Next is the **barbell tricep crossover**.

While lying flat on the bench hold the barbell in your right hand (facing outward) parallel to the chest. Bend the forearm at the elbow, positioning barbell approximately two inches over the left side of chest. Raise barbell back to starting position repeating rotation for a minimum of three sets. Switch barbell to the left hand and duplicate same routine. The last exercise for triceps is called **kickbacks**.

While bending forward and holding selected barbell in right hand, position left foot in front of you and right foot to your rear. Hold barbell in front of you with arm bent at elbow. Bend the knees slightly and proceed to extend forearm outward toward rear. Return to starting position and repeat rotation a minimum of three sets. Left hand position should have right foot forward, left foot toward rear. Repeat same rotation.

Day Two (2) Back and Upper Deltoids:

We will start with **one-arm barbell rows** better known as lawn mowers. This exercise will focus on the lateral area of the back. Position the selected barbell on the floor next to a weight bench. Place your left hand and knee on the bench; grab the barbell with your right hand and pull toward your chest. Return back to your starting position without touching the floor with the weight. Repeat this rotation for a minimum of three sets.

The second exercise for the back will be **bent over rows** with the straight bar. Start by placing both feet parallel to your shoulders. Knees should be slightly bent to prevent shifting.

Arch the lower back to reduce the risk of injury to it. While in this position grab the bar right outside of your feet. Begin pulling the bar upward above the abdomen and below the chest. Continue this motion being sure that you isolate the upper back when you pull inward and stretching when you release. Repeat for a minimum of three sets.

The third exercise will be **lateral rows** to focus on expanding the lateral area. This routine, incorporated with some great core routines, will help to create a total V shape. Start By connecting one of the straight bars to the cable machine. Place your hands on the bar extended about shoulder length. Begin pulling the bar in a downward position over your knee area. Return to the extended position and repeat rotation. Four reps are recommended simply because this is one of the key areas for creating width and depth.

Day Three (3) Shoulders:

This first exercise is your basic seated dumbbell **shoulder press.** Using two dumbbells while seated on a bench raise both arms being sure they both are parallel to one another at your sides. Once you are ready push the weight in an upright position when the arms are extended begin contracting your shoulders.

The second exercise is **outside flies.** Your weight should be decreased because it may be harder to use the same weight as used in the overhead press since it is harder to raise the arms toward the sides than it is to lift overhead. Therefore, using a lighter weight is an alternative. Now, once prepared, take the arms, hold them up in almost the same position as used in the overhead press except the arms are placed toward the front of the body. Gradually bring the arms upward, keeping them at your sides being sure the elbow is higher than the fist when raised.

Then lower your arms back to start position. Repeat the motion for three sets and as many reps as is desired goal.

Lastly, for day three, the third exercise **front raises** can be used with the same weight as used with **outside flies**. Start by holding the arms dropped at your sides and the barbells in both right and left hands. Your knuckles should be facing frontward. Gradually raise your arms extended in front of you until they are about eye level. Once at this position isolate the shoulder area as much as possible. This is the complete rotation needed now lower the arms and repeat the motion for three sets and as many reps necessary to achieve desired goal.

Day Four (4) cardiovascular drills and core routines:

Cardio will consist of 20 minutes on the treadmill.

For the first ten minutes the speed will be rotated every two minutes. Example= if your low point is 3.4 after two minutes your speed will be changed to 5.4 then reduced after two minutes is complete. Next will be 15 minutes on the elliptical machine

Once the cardio workout is complete we then proceed to our core routines. The first exercise for core will be **windmills.** This is one of the best ways to draw the upper core into the lateral area. Using a body bar or pole across the shoulders will help to not only isolate the core but aid in maintaining form. Be sure not to pull down on the bar it simply used as a guide. Once the bar is placed on the shoulders spread your arms across the bar and your feet wide. Begin turning your body at the waste from right to left. Upon each turn be sure to isolate the obliques and keep the feet as stationary as possible. Higher repetitions would be sufficient for this routine.

Second exercise **Hanging knee raises**

For this particular routine you can use the harness if one is available. Place your arms in at the elbows holding the straps at the top. Once you are in position let the body hang and then begin raising your knees toward your chest. Allow the knees to drop and then repeat the rotation. Upon doing core routines higher repetitions are always better.

Third exercise **laying crunches**

To start position yourself on your back with your legs erect place the hands behind your head and begin raising your upper body. Each time the upper body is raised contract your core as much as possible. Lower your self without completely resting the shoulders on the floor then repeat rotation. Crunch for as many repetitions as you can endure be sure not to add pressure on the neck or back.

Day Five (5) Legs

First we start with your basic squat this exercise can be done several ways depending on your level of training. Starting with the straight bar placed over the shoulders. The feet can be position inside of the elbows and outside of the shoulders. Slightly bend the knees and arch the lower back to help reduce the risk of injury. Now you can begin squatting slowly with your feet planted firmly to the floor. Return to a standing position without locking or snapping the knees at the joints.

Second exercise **Hamstring machine.**

Set the key to the desired weight lay down on the bench and place your feet with both heels under the pads and begin raising the bar toward your hamstring. After this is done extend the feet back to its starting position then repeat for 3 sets.

Third exercise **Calves machine.**

By using the calf machine raise your heals and isolate the calve area so that   the tension is felt on the targeted muscle. Repeat for 3 sets.

You now have a five-day workout regimen with three exercises for each muscle group that can be rotated as you please. You can also use it for as long as you like because the weights can be adjust according to your training level. Modifications can be made for beginners by substituting weights for cable cross over or smith machines.

Chapter 4

Five-day Diet Plan

Day (1) **Breakfast** – One small bowl of hot multi grain cereal, Barley or oat. 1 green apple and two egg whites, may add one glass of water or natural tea.

Day (1) **Lunch** – one sandwich with natural almond butter and natural blue berry jam on whole wheat. 1 slice of melon 1 stick of celery and 1 whey or casein protein shake. Water may be added to reduce the calorie intake.

Day (1) **Dinner** – A slice of salmon a fair portion of broccoli and a small portion of whole-wheat pasta. And 1 glass of fresh water.

Your first days diet consist of low carbohydrates whole-wheat protein vitamin C and E

Day (2) **Breakfast** – 1 hot bowl of cream of rice cereal 2 slices of rye toast 2 slice of pineapple 1 glass of fresh water.

Day (2) **Lunch** – Tuna salad and artichoke with Whole-wheat crackers and 1 carrot. May add one glass of fresh water.

Day (2) **Dinner** – 1 Turkey breast, brown basmati long grained rice and spinach. May add fresh water.

Day (3) Breakfast- Kashi Go Lean Crunch, or other high fiber cereal, 2 slices of whole wheat bread, and one banana. May add fresh water.

Day (3) Lunch- 1 piece of chicken breast, wheat pasta and fruit salad, flax seed and 1 whey protein shake.

Day (3) Dinner- 1 Trout fish, 1 full salad with low fat dressing, black beans and sliced Almonds. May add one glass fresh water.

Day (4) Breakfast- peanut butter and apple jam on whole wheat bread or toast, low fat yogurt and sliced pears. May add one glass fresh water.

Day (4) Lunch- turkey sandwich on rye or wheat bread, 2 carrots, 2 celery stalks, 1 red apple and 1 glass of whey protein shake. May add fresh water.

Day (4) Dinners- Stuffed cabbage rolls of lean ground turkey wrapped in layers with long grain rice and spinach. May add fresh water.

Day (5) Breakfast- 1 bowl of oat meal, 1 muffin with jam and wolf berries which are high in antioxidants and can also act as an immune booster.

Day (5) Lunch- 1 helping of egg salad, 1 whey protein shake and broccoli which contains many vitamins, high in vitamin C and E and packed with antioxidants.

Day (5) Dinner- Whole wheat Egg noodles, 1 chicken breast, and smothered tomatoes that also contains powerful antioxidants such as lycopene. When cooked more antioxidants are released.

All portions should consist of small meals because they are healthier for the digestive system.

The meals listed in this weekly diet plan consist of fat burning products, natural carbohydrates and whole grains as well as foods that are found to be super foods.

Based on some studies the following foods are found to be highly effective in promoting great health.

Avocados-rich in vitamin C, aids in the digestive system and may improve the skin.

Garlic- helps to thin the blood. Also may prevent blood clots heart attacks and strokes.

Broccoli- high in antioxidants vitamin C and E, as well as many other vitamins.

Tomatoes - also contains many antioxidants.

Blue berries- another source of antioxidants, fiber, calcium vitamin A and C. Studies suggests that that they can also aid eye sight.

Wolfberries- are strong antioxidants-which may boost the immune system and contains 500 times more vitamins c than oranges. Also rich in amino acids with large amounts of b2 and b6 as well as beta carotene

Sardines -which is rich in Omega3 and protein

Kale- high in fiber, iron and calcium

Spinach- very high in nutrients

Tea- Green or Black

Chapter 5

Reducing Body Fat

You can reduce your body fat by maintaining a calorie-restricted diet along with exercise to build muscle. You can practice eating foods that will not only aid in fat burning but will help muscle growth. The diet that I have recommended in the weekly diet plan will help aid in supporting the digestive system. Diet is also important in creating a healthy flow of the arteries there-for preventing clogging. Clogging is one of the main causes of heart attaché. Monitoring a healthy diet is a key factor in staying fit. This applies to people with or without health issues. People that suffer from diabetes, high or low blood pressure, heart decease, fibromyalgia and many other ailments will benefit greatly from diet and exercise. We have more power over the quality of our health than we realize it is a God given gift called will. This not only applies to how you look but how you feel, think and perform. Be mindful that eliminating body fat and body weight are in-fact two different things. Men with more than 20% body fat are over fat, and woman with more than 30% body fat are over fat. Over weight simply means that you are more than 10% percent of your ideal weight. Below is a body fat chart of maximum recommended percentage based on many studies.

Refer to "Body Fat Charts."

Body Fat Charts

Women

Age	Excellent	Good	Fair	Poor
20-24	18.9	22.0	25.0	29.6
25-29	18.9	22.1	25.4	29.8
30-34	19.7	22.7	26.4	30.5
35-39	21.0	24.0	27.7	31.5
40-44	22.6	25.6	29.3	32.8
45-49	24.3	27.3	30.9	34.1
50-54	26.2	29.7	33.1	36.2
60+	27.6	31.0	24.1	38.0

Men

Age	Excellent	Good	Fair	Poor
20-24	10.8	14.9	19.0	23.3
25-29	12.8	16.5	20.3	24.3
30-34	14.5	18.0	21.5	25.2
35-39	16.1	19.3	22.6	26.1
40-44	17.5	20.5	23.6	26.9
45-49	18.6	21.5	24.5	27.6
50-54	19.8	22.7	25.6	28.7
60+	20.3	23.5	26.7	29.8

Chapter 6

Breathing Techniques

There are no specific regulations in reference to breathing during fitness training. Although it is found that circulating your breathing during cardio or weight training is very helpful. Allowing air to go in through the nose and out of mouth helps to circulate breathing. When the lungs are filled with too much air at one time you can begin to hyperventilate. It might feel as though you have a huge ball of cotton in your throat. Breathing in deep through the nose and holding it for about five seconds and then releasing it through the mouth will help to slow your heart rate. This will also give better opportunity for controlled breathing. It is very important to monitor your body during training. By listening to your body you will be able to notice any signs of trouble. Providing you have any heart trouble you should consult your physician before considering training of any sort. If you notice any chest pains arising you should stop training immediately and seek medical or professional help. Learning to breath can push your endurance and allow you to perform under shorter intervals. By conditioning your lungs to support a deeper wind span will allow more air there-for creating more oxygen. While pushing against the force of the weight you can exhale and inhale when releasing. For example if you where using the flat bench for chest you would exhale when pushing the weight up and inhale

when lowering the weight. It is important to practice great
breathing techniques because it can help prevent hemorrhoids,
hernias, or dizziness.

Chapter 7

Recommendations for Protein Intake

The best time to exercise your protein intake is the first thing in the morning and the last thing at night. Before sleeping to help support protein breakdown and when you wake because your protein levels are down because of lack of food intake during sleep. It is suggested that you should digest at least 9 grams of protein per lean pound of body weight. New studies by the international journal of sports nutrition suggest that people involved in strength training need 7 grams per pound. You want to be sure that the body remain in a muscle building state. For example a 200-pound man (200* .7) would need 140 grams of protein. Upon taking protein supplements you can also add the fruit papaya because it will also aid in supporting the digestive system. The better a protein is absorbed by the body the higher the BV level will be. Below is a chart of the biological value of some foods.

Protein	BV
Whey Isolate	110-159
Whey Concentrate	104
Whole Egg	100
Cow's milk	91
Egg white	88
Fish	83
Beef	80
Chicken	79
Casein	77
Soy	74
Rice	59
Wheat	54
Beans	49

Chapter 8

Recommended Juice Combinations for Health

Subject to our busy schedules, practicing a healthy diet is difficult. However, there are simple options to finding and preparing meals that provide the necessary nutrients the body needs. Having a juice machine at home is a vital tool to improve the quality of our lives. There are many nutritious meals that can be made that can assist in preventing and treating several health issues. Below are just a few combinations:

Blood Pressure: carrot, celery, parsley, spinach, tomatoes

Colds: carrot, spinach, orange, ginger

Diabetes: lemon, carrot, parsley, and celery

Digestive system: Red apple, carrot, beet, lemon, ginger

Gastritis: carrot, apple, cucumber, cabbage

Liver support: apple, carrot, celery

Arthritis: spinach juice, parsley juice, cucumber

Asthma: carrot juice, spinach juice, parsley juice

Bladder ailments: carrot juice, beet juice, cucumber, dandelion

Ginseng Shake: 5-year-old ginger root in apple juice with blended banana and honey

Total affect: one ounce of fresh wheat grass

Chapter 9

Stress Reduction

Some symptoms of stress may be physical or psychological. Illnesses such as irritable bowel syndrome, heart attacks, high blood pressure, and chronic headaches can occur. Major changes such as job loss, divorce, or completing ones education may also have some psychological effects. Stress can also break down the immune system and make the body susceptible to virus. Physical training offers options.

Fitness can help strengthen the body, reduce stress and create a defense mechanism to help fight off virus. Practicing a healthy diet will help cleanse and relieve the body of toxins. This may also reflect on how you feel and function while performing your daily life activities. We must remember the importance of supporting our bodies in its ability to regulate and reject impurities. This rule applies even for today's vegetarians because of the insecticides used on crop to prevent contamination from pestilence.

Chronic stress or long term stress may not allow the body to return to a relaxed state. Instead of boosting the immune system, chronic stress appears to slow the immune feedback. This increases the risk of infection and affects the response to immunization. Acute stress activates the natural defense system this can result in boosting the immune system temporarily.

Exercise, walking or jogging, are all great methods of stress reduction. 8-10 hours of sleep regularly, eating healthy, social activities with friends and research are also great tools that may be used.

Chapter 10

Warm-up Routine

This is a warm up routine that can be used daily. In it you will notice that it will not only stress your cardiovascular system but will cut your cardio time in half. For the more advanced individual, jumping rope is advised. There are also several tricks that you may learn to keep jumping from being too repetitious or dull. As your endurance builds you can utilize the clock adding an extra two minutes and shortening the time of your intermission between sets creating faster intervals. For the less advanced individual, there is the treadmill or elliptical machine. When using these machines you can monitor the clock taking note where your low number is so that you may rotate your meter to push your endurance level as well as cutting your cardio in half. For example, if your low number is 3.0 after walking at that pace for a warm up when ready you can change the speedometer to 4.4 for an entire minute. When the last two digits on the clock read .00 a minute has passed. You should then return the meter to 3.0. This should be repeated at a minimum of 4 times before returning to a consistent pace (considered a sprint). Each time you return to the gym you should add an extra point on the meter also an extra sprint. So instead of 3.0 to start you are at 4.0 and your high number would become 5.5. Utilizing this technique 15-20 minutes should

be great therefore giving more time for weight training.

Chapter 11

Weekly Home Workout Plan

* Note: Each exercise should be done a minimum of 3 sets with reps of 12-15.

Day One - Chest and Triceps

1st exercise- this is simply a modification to simulate the weekly gym work out that was given. Although this workout can be done at home it is still effective in getting great results. For the less experienced trainee this push up chest routine can be done on the knees while leaning against a wall. Be sure to isolate and contract the muscle so that the blood is directed toward the targeted muscle group. 4 sets of 12-15 to begin are good. If you can endure more it is okay to extend yourself.

2nd exercise- now we can move on to diamond push-ups. This routine will not only give more peak to the chest muscles but will also contract the secondary muscle, which is the triceps. Place both hands close together with the fingers pointed toward each other creating a diamond shaped position. You will find that it is a bit easier to contract the chest muscle in this position. 4 sets of 12-15 are good for this routine also.

3rd exercise- now we move to push ups with the hands turned outward as if in a wing handed position. Keep the arms pressed closely to your sides to create more isolation on the triceps muscle.

Day Two - Back and Upper Deltoids

1st exercise- Bent over flies. While seated on the edge of a chair using two soup cans bend over slightly. Once in this position raise the arm behind you being sure to lead with your elbows. Repeat this motion for 12-15 reps.

2nd exercise- Standing flies. This routine can also be done with two, 15oz. soup cans. Hold the cans out to your sides. When ready bring the cans forward in front of you and then rotate your hand behind you in a raised position. Be sure to isolate the back and upper deltoids when your arms are toward the rear of you. (See note above)

3rd exercise- One Arm Rows. This exercise can be done with a slightly heavier prop. A bottle of 32 oz. detergent can be utilized. With one hand and knee placed against a chair bend over slightly allowing the arm holding the bottle to hang. Lift the bottle upward isolating the lateral area of your back.

Day 3- Shoulders

1st exercise- Overhead shoulder press. Using two, 15oz. Soup cans, one in each hand, raise arms to a 45-degree angle and parallel to each other simultaneously and begin to push upward. Return to starting position and repeat motion.

2nd exercise- Outside flies. Using the two soup cans as props hold them both in front of you with your elbows slightly bent. Then begin to raise your arms at the elbows above your shoulders. Repeat this motion as suggested in note.

3rd exercise- Front flies. Using the same props, hold cans to your sides and begin raising them in front of you to eye level. Return to your starting position and repeat motion.

Day Four- Cardio and Core

1st exercise- Rowing toe touches. Begin by holding your arms raised out toward your sides. As you reach from right to left and reverse touch your toes. This can be done for 15-20 minutes with only 20-second intermissions.

2nd exercise- Windmills. Can be done with your arms spread wide. Once in this position begin to turn the body from right to left and left to right. Isolate the core throughout the entire range of motion. Repeat for 4 sets of 15-20. Also, be mindful that right to left is one rep. This is how the rotation should be counted to be sure that the exercise is completed for a rotation.

3rd exercise- Crunches. This exercise can be done while lying on the floor. To be sure that the neck is protected you can place the hands behind the neck as you begin to raise the upper body in a crunch position. Do not pull the head up adding pressure on the neck. The hands are simply used as a guide. Repeat sets as suggested in note with 20-second intermissions.

4th exercise- Side rows. Stand with your arms at your sides. When positioned, begin bending to the right side, then to the left, acting as if you are reaching for the floor. Repeat as suggested in note.

Day Five- Legs

1st exercise- Squats. This exercise can be done using natural body weight. Be sure to keep the lower back arched and the heels rooted to the floor. While in the squat position be sure your head remains over your knees and does not exceed your feet. Repeat as suggested in note with 20-second intermissions.

2nd exercise- Lunges. Start in an upright position. Begin taking one step forward touching each knee on the floor in front of you one at a time. Complete as suggested in note with no intermission.

3rd exercise- Side lunges. Your starting position is an upright stance. Begin by stepping to your right side while bending the knee in a squatting position. Repeat the motion stepping next to the left side. Repeat as suggested in note with 20-second intermissions.

Chapter 12

Obesity Amongst Youth

Obesity amongst children in the united state is growing at a rapid rate 1 out of 3 kids suffer from obesity. Television, computers and video games play a major roll in limiting a child's activities. Fast foods and a lack of nutritional home cooked meals play an even greater roll. Parents may incorporate fun sport activities in their family pass time events such as basketball, football, baseball, jump rope, jogging, racing, etc. They're are forms of cardio vascular exercises which gets the heart rate pumping and also increasing one's metabolism. Plenty of exercise will also create healthy stamina strength and flexibility. If you believe that your child is overweight you can review the body mass index (BMI) this formula uses height and weight measurements to estimate how much body fat a person has. One should consult a physician before attempting to determine what the body weight or body fat of a child should be. To prevent obesity a healthy diets can be prepared for children just as adults, Complex carbohydrates, vegetables, whole grains and proteins. Calcium consists of low fat milk, cottage cheese and yogurt. Proteins such as fresh meats, chicken, lean beef or grilled fish are also great. Great sources of vegetables are broccoli, spinach or asparagus, which contain vitamins A, C, K and several B vitamins. We must regain control over the influence that our children have pertaining to there diets. One of the best ways of doing this is getting back to family dinners. It seems as though today's busy schedules' have kept us from sharing this important event there-for subjecting us to fast foods most times unhealthy for us. If your daily activities don't allow time or the energy to prepare a home cook meal we can choose to dine out with our children at which a healthy dining selection can still be made. This not only encourages good eating habits but it allows for quality bonding time with family. This act is so very important because it gives us an even greater opportunity to get to know and understand our children. Through bonding our children are more likely to confide in family at times of need be for there peers. It is most often through the love and advise of family that our youth develop good decision making skills. This entire analogy may show how through fitness and dieting healthy life style skills can be produced. When you feel good you think good and out of good thoughts come good actions. When a child practices health consciousness he or she can be less likely to do things that are harmful to there body. This may help in the area of drug prevention or anything else that may be harmful for them.

Chapter 13

Acknowledgements

I would first love to thank God who has given me the passion and knowledge that I may give to others. Health is one of the greatest gifts that God has granted us. With out it we have very little. Our physical and emotional wellness can depend on the condition of our health. As a kid my mother instilled in me the importance of physical well being. When my mother was pregnant with my younger sister, people would ask her, "What would you like to give birth to, girl or boy?" My mother would respond, "during the birth of my children, the first thing I do is count the fingers and toes, pray for total health, then thank God for a healthy baby. That's all that matters." To my stepfather, who instilled in me the importance of hard work, thank you. And to my four beautiful sisters who placed me in a position to be motivated enough to work out so that I could be their protector.

Today I have a position in society as a mentor and boxing trainer. This keeps me motivated to maintain health consciousness because I want to be an example to others. To every one who has motivated and encouraged me in the area of diet and fitness, I am highly appreciative. To Carmine, owner and proprietor of Gold Coast Gym, one of the greatest gyms in Jersey City, I say thanks for your support. Also, I wish plenty of success for the USA Boxing Association and all of their coaches. To all of the professional and amateur fighters that I have had the pleasure to work with, keep up the good work! And to my client and good friend David Kay who has been very supportive, thank you as well. Lastly, thanks to all of the churches in the city that has allowed me to utilize their space to conduct workshops and mentor.

Appendix

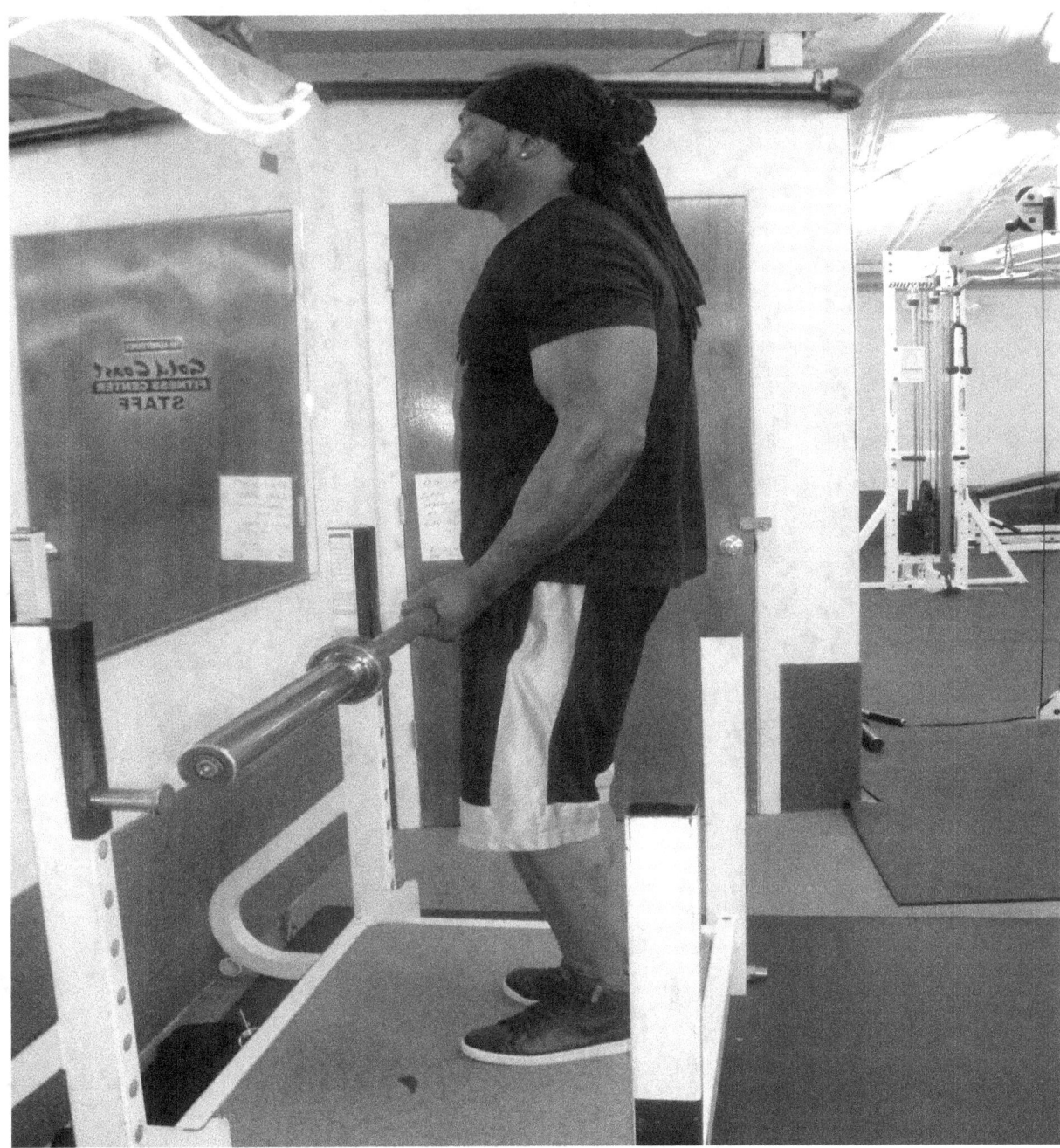

Warm-up straight bar curl 1

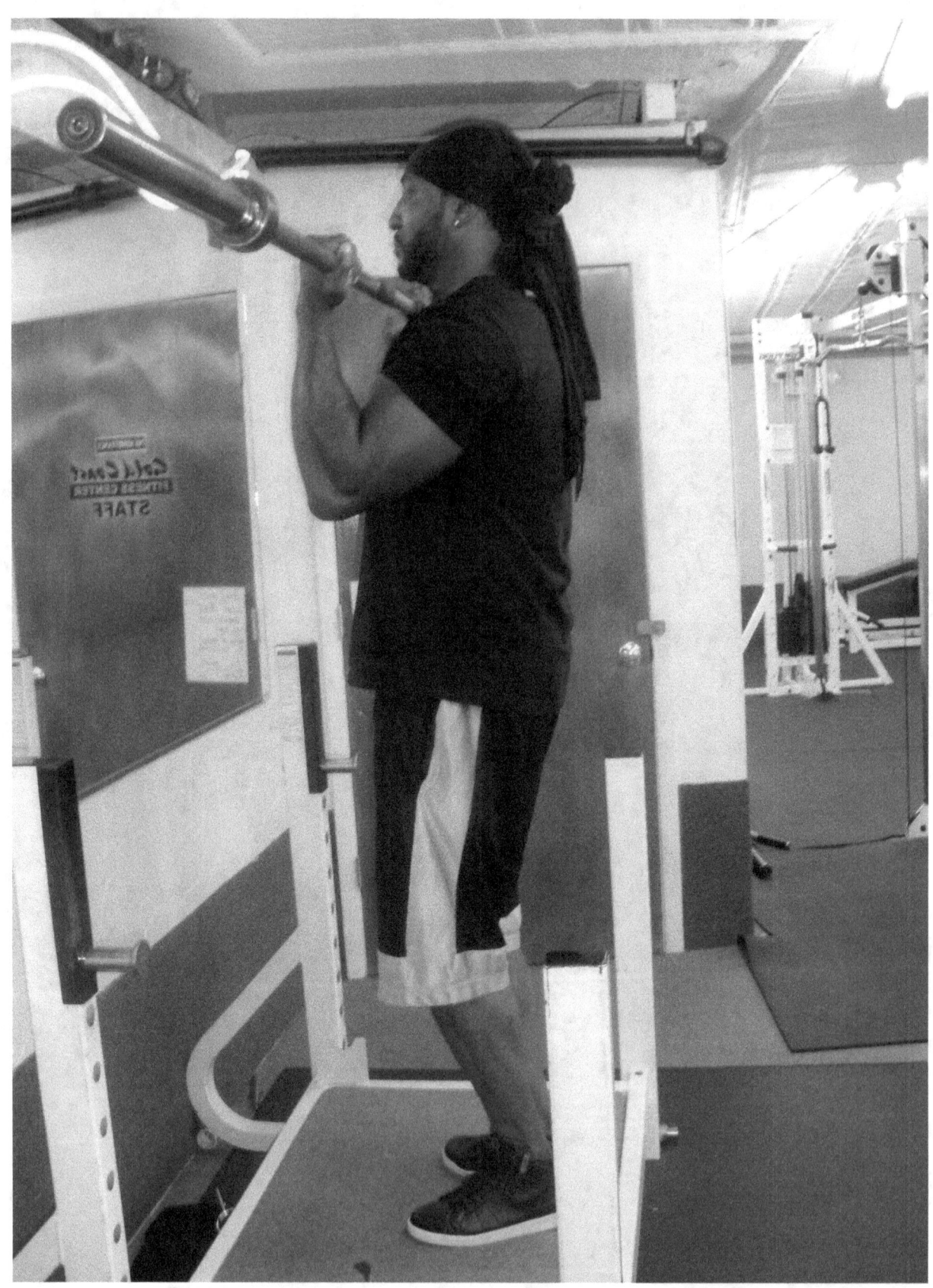

Warm-up straight bar curl 2

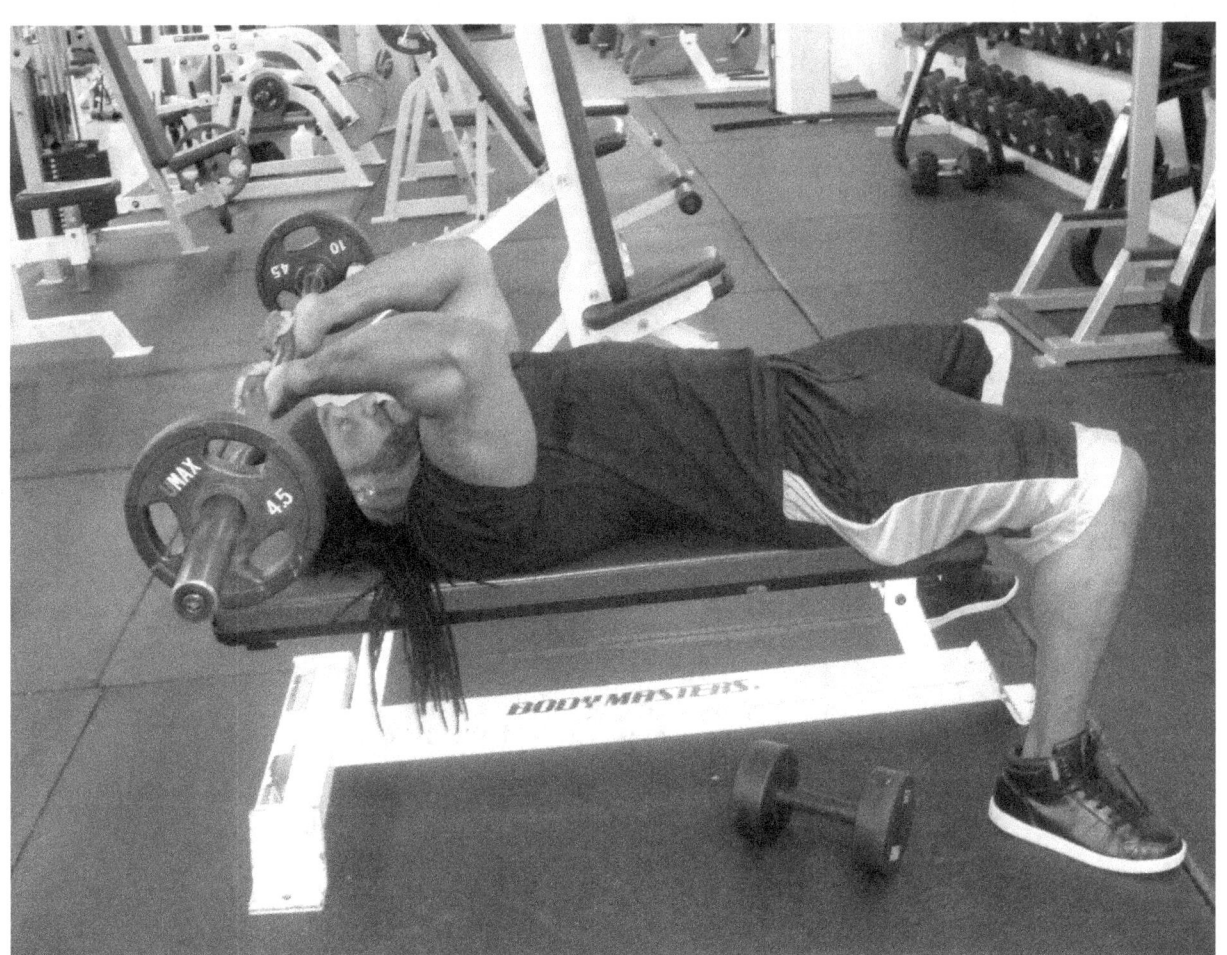

Straight-bar triceps press 1

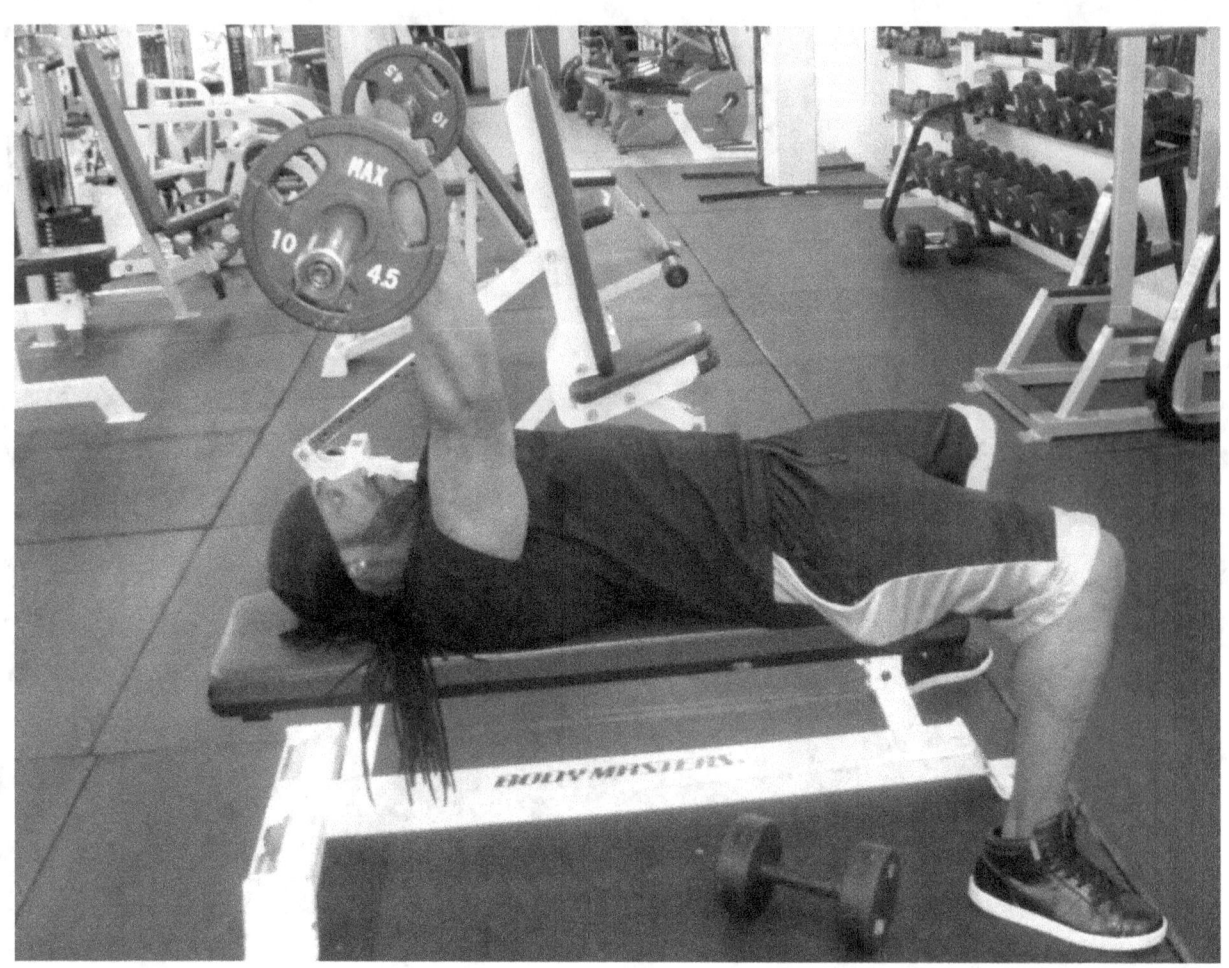

Straight-bar triceps press 2

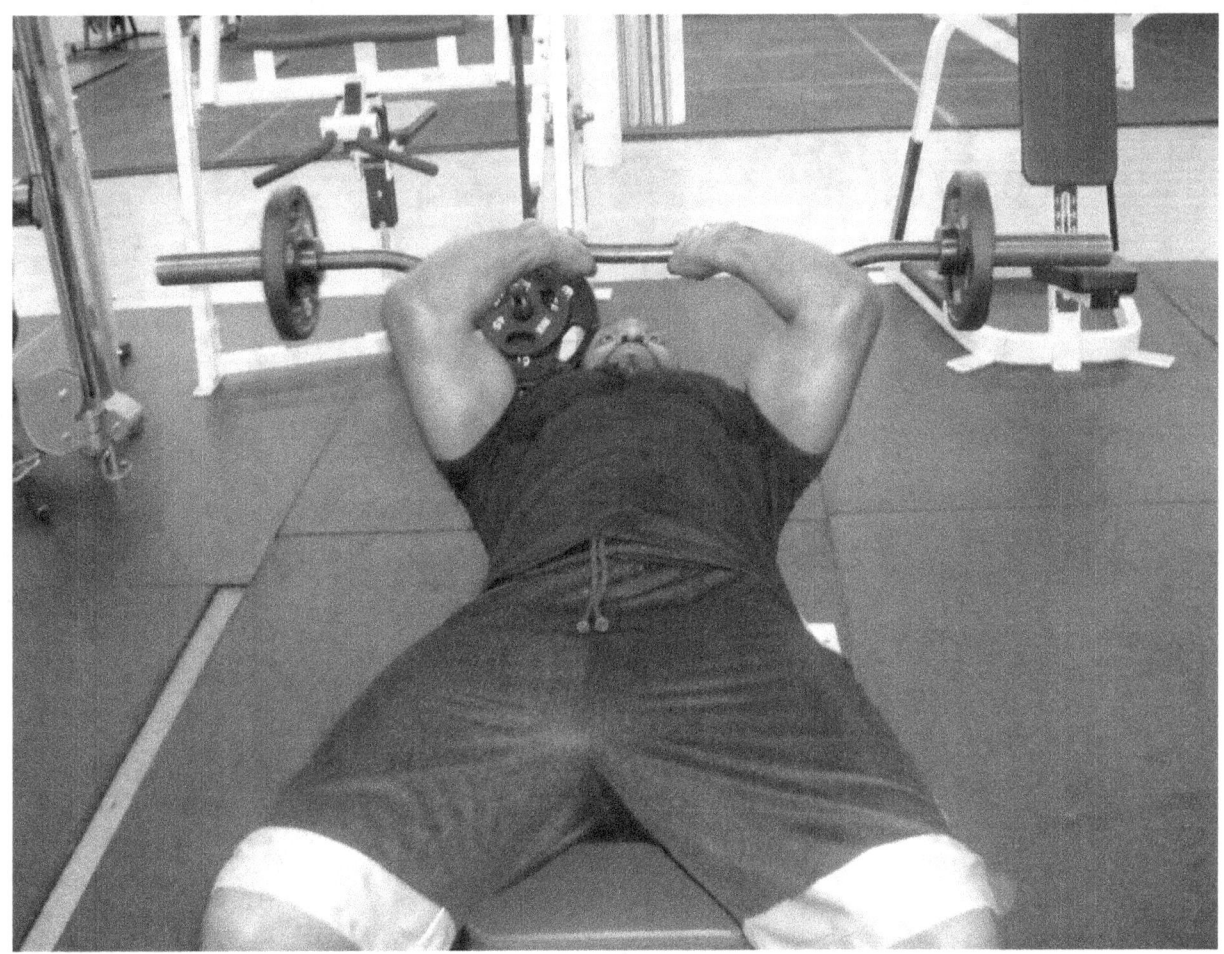

Curl bar triceps press

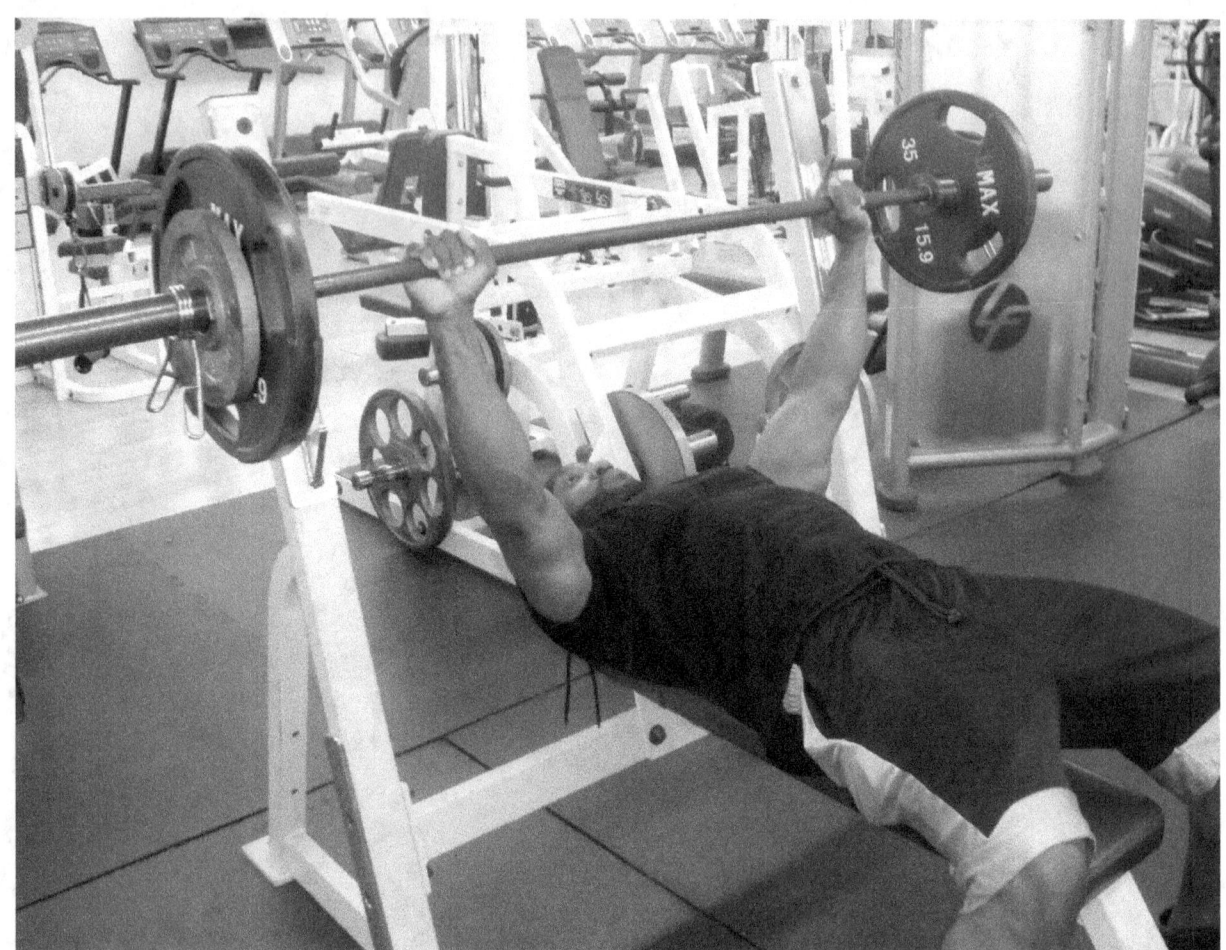

Flat bench 1

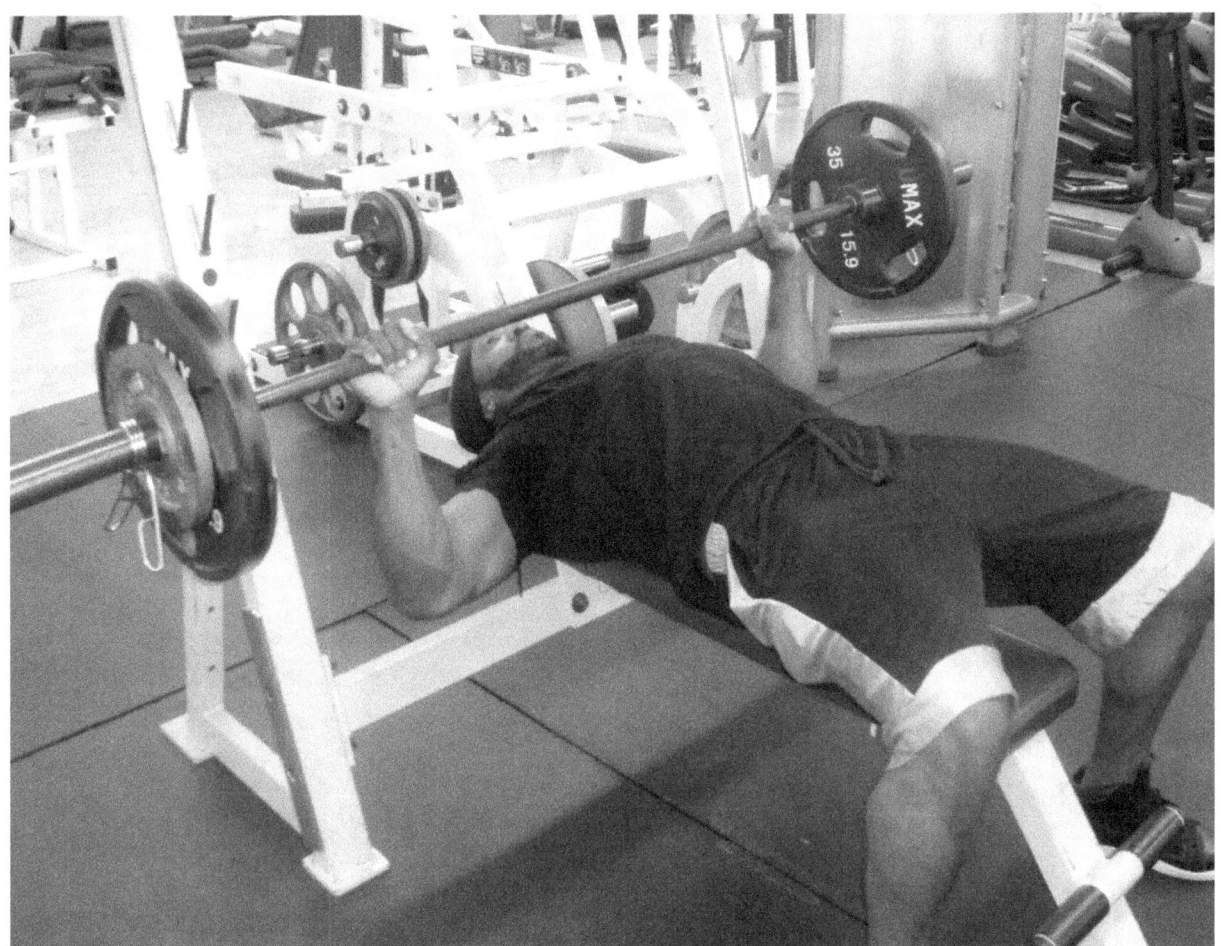

Flat bench 2

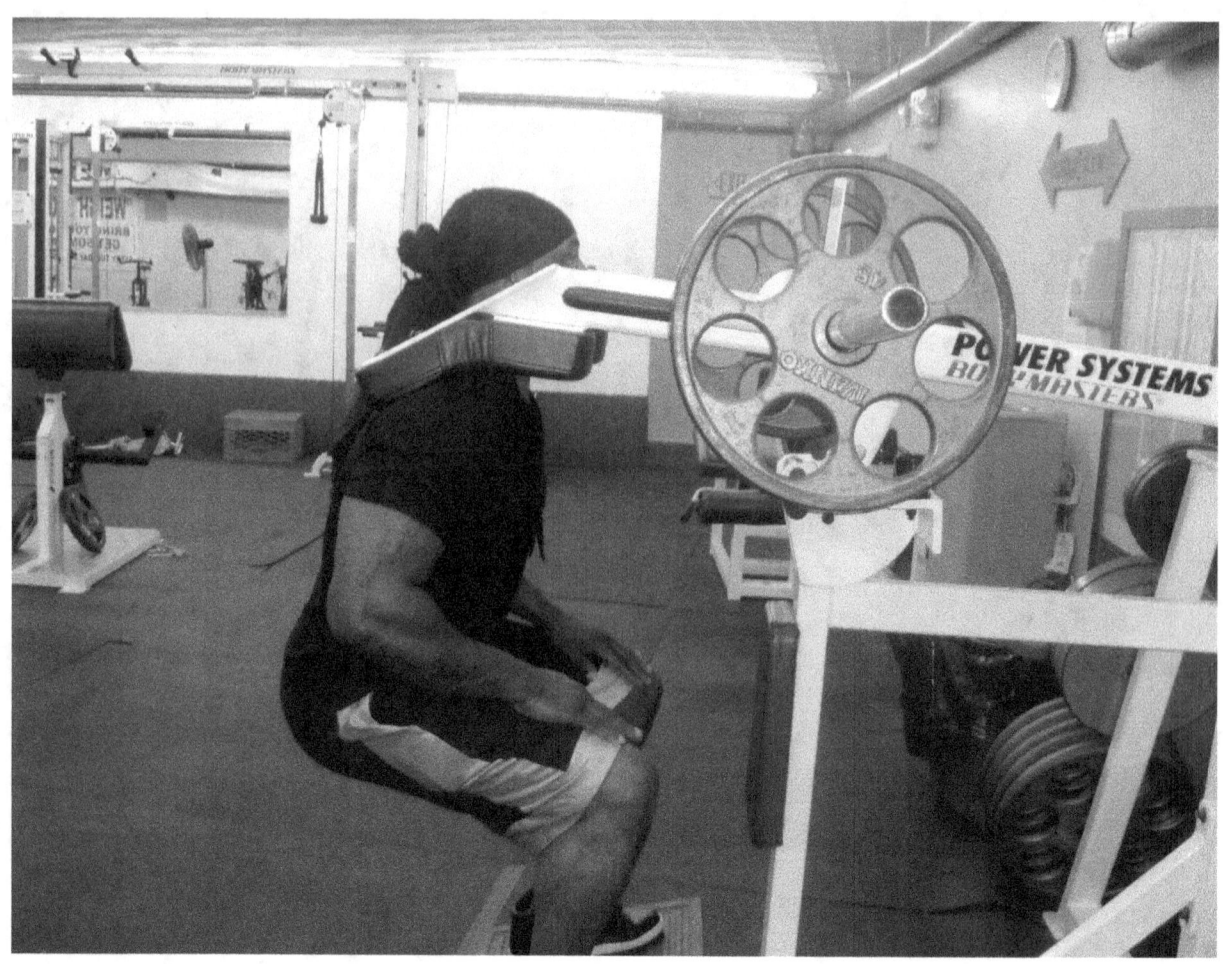

Squat press

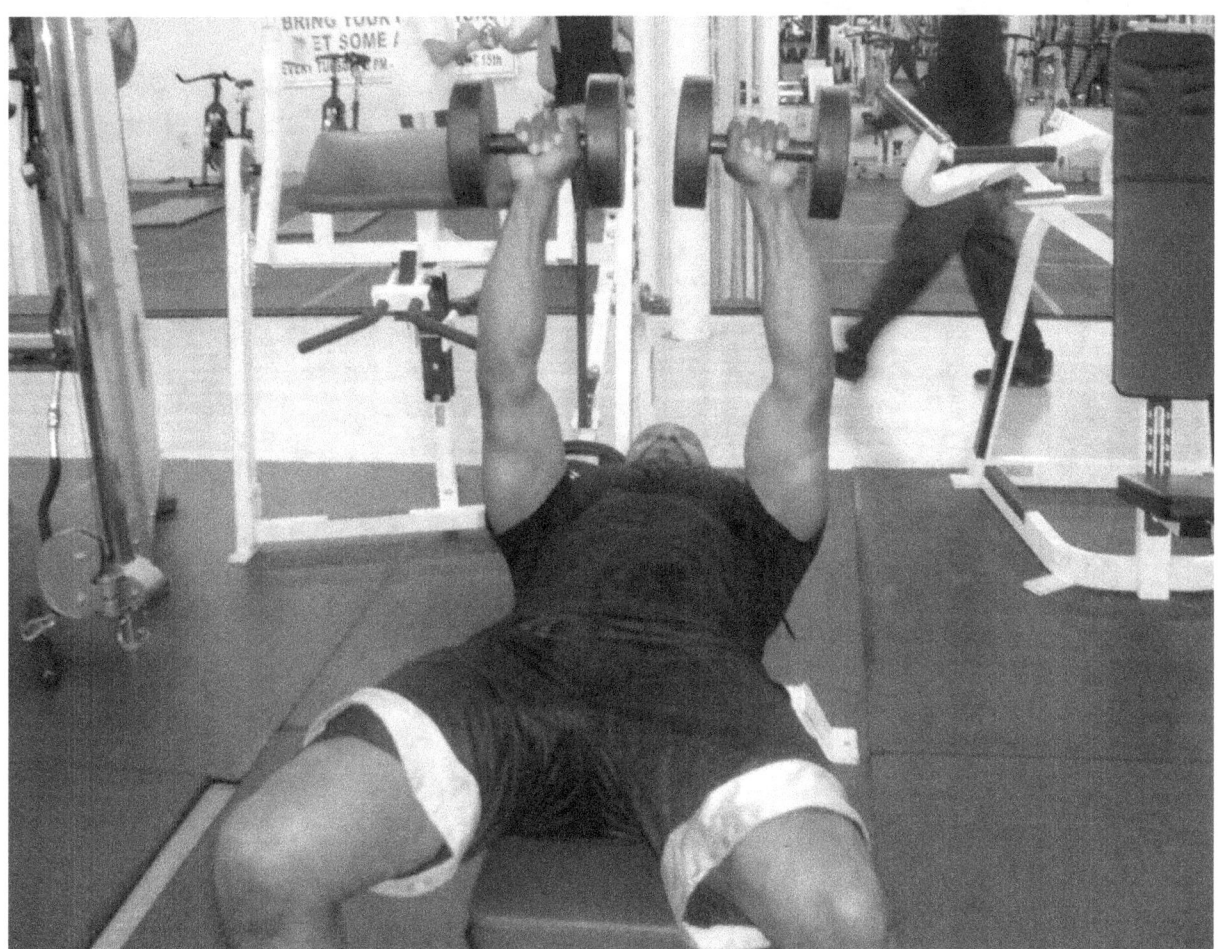

Dumbbell chest press 1

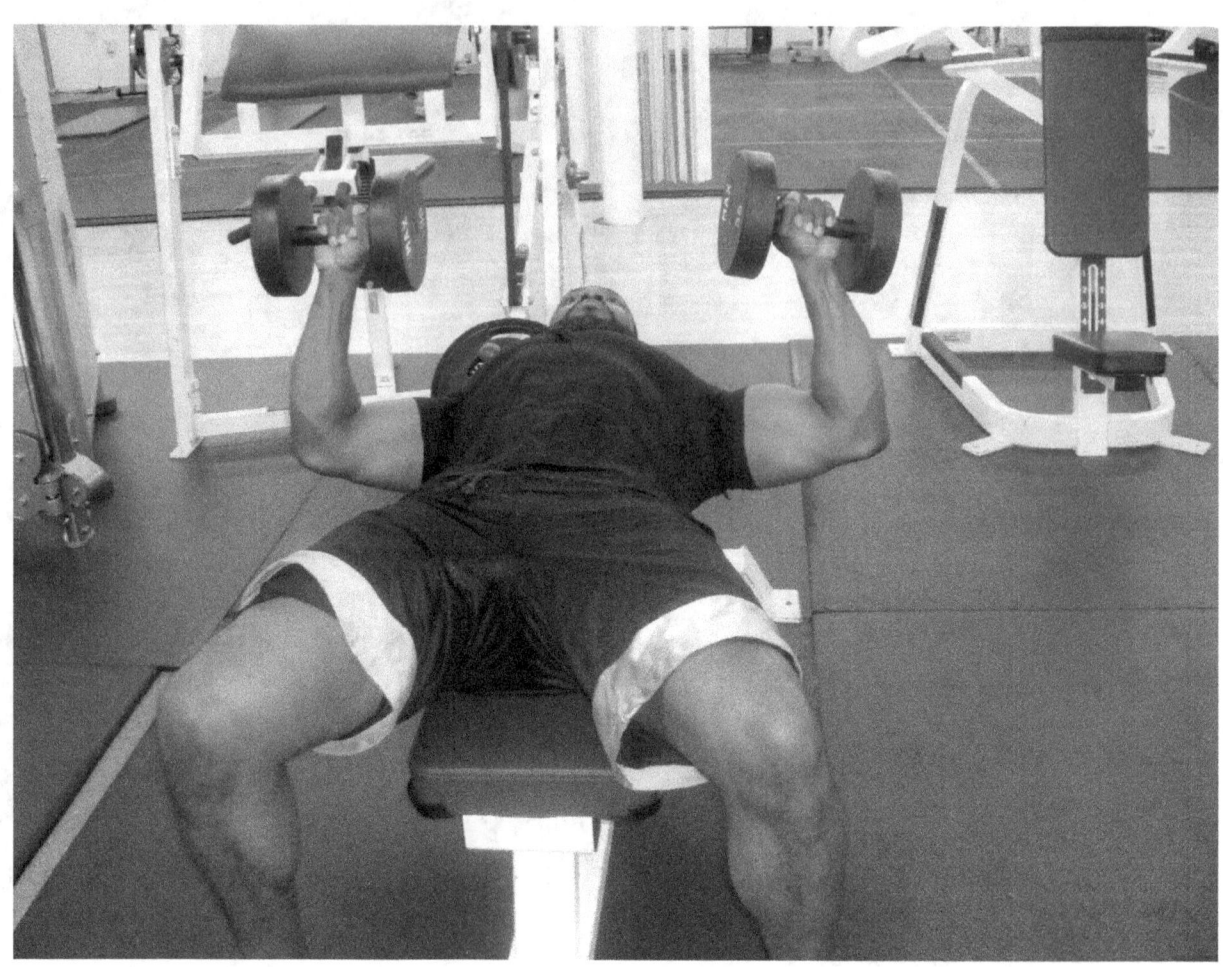

Dumbbell chest press 2

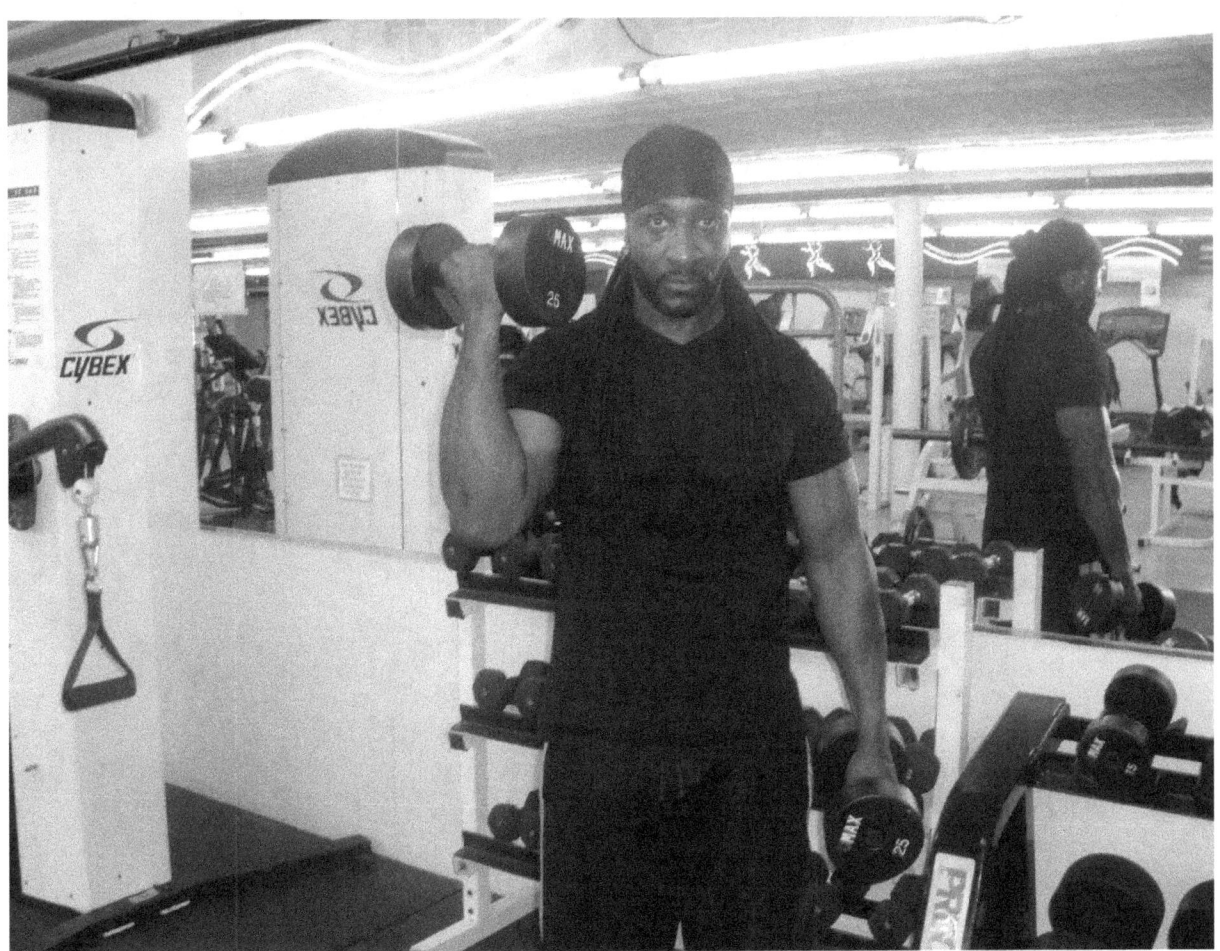

Dumbbell curl 1

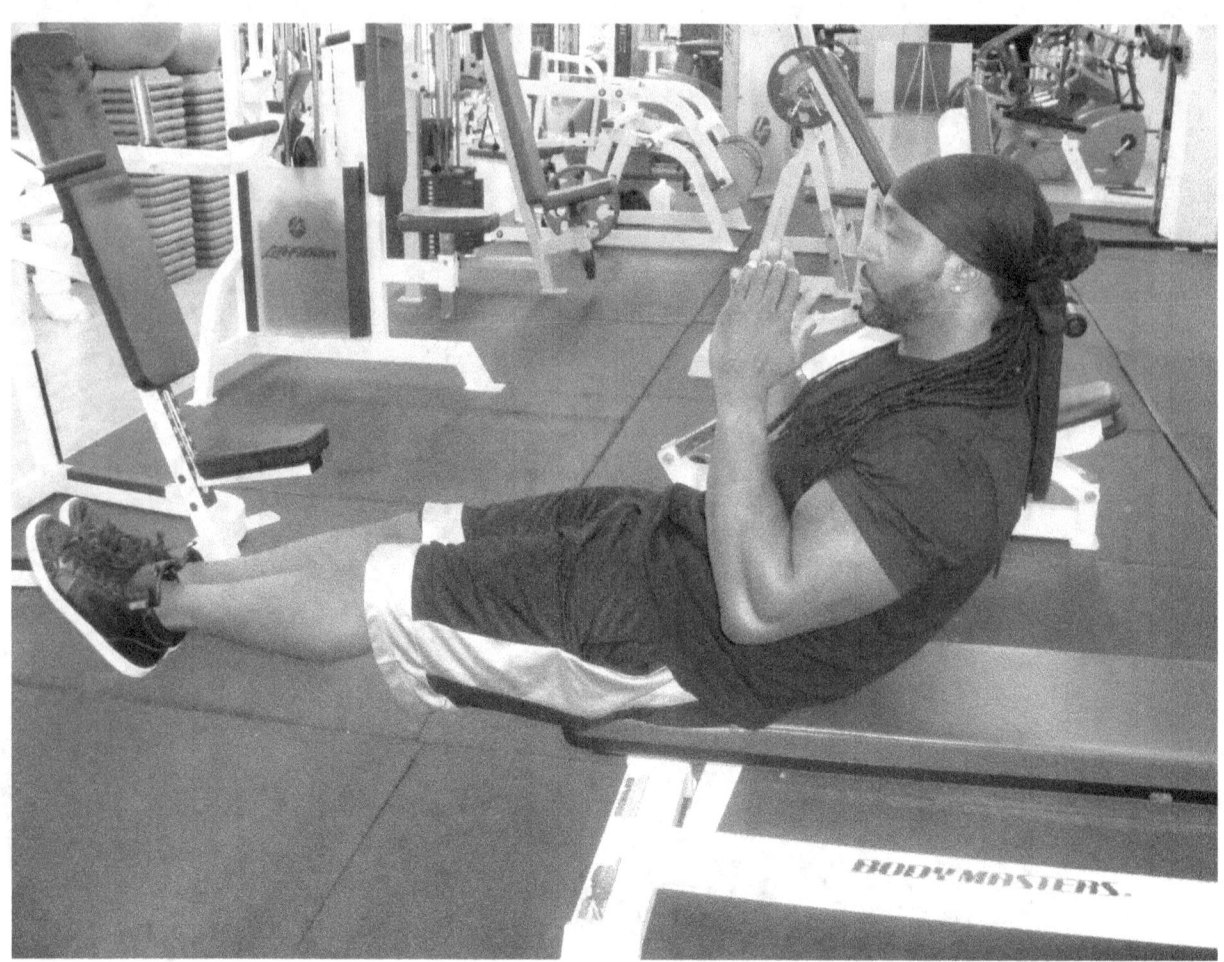

Knee raise crunch 1

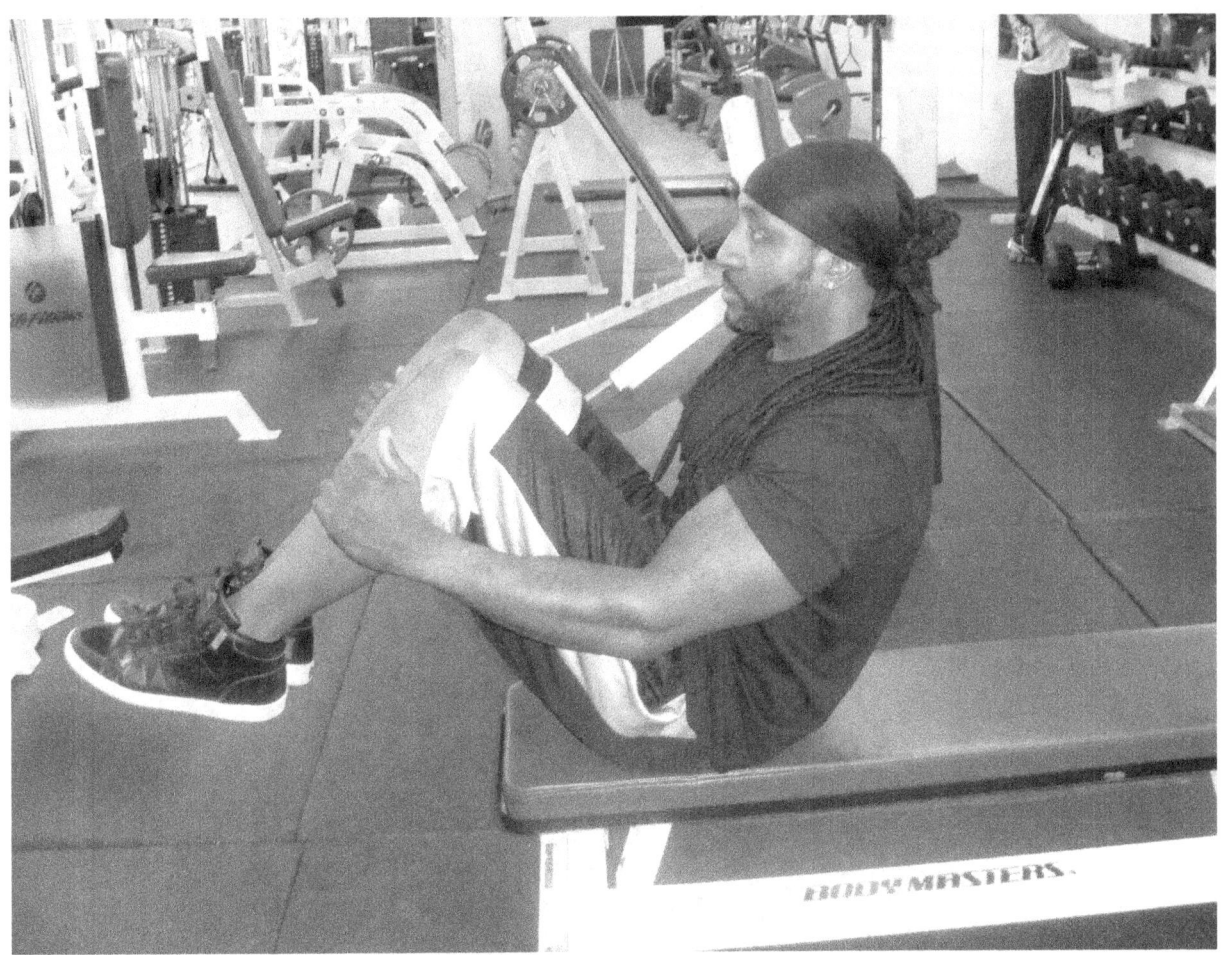

Knee raise crunch 2

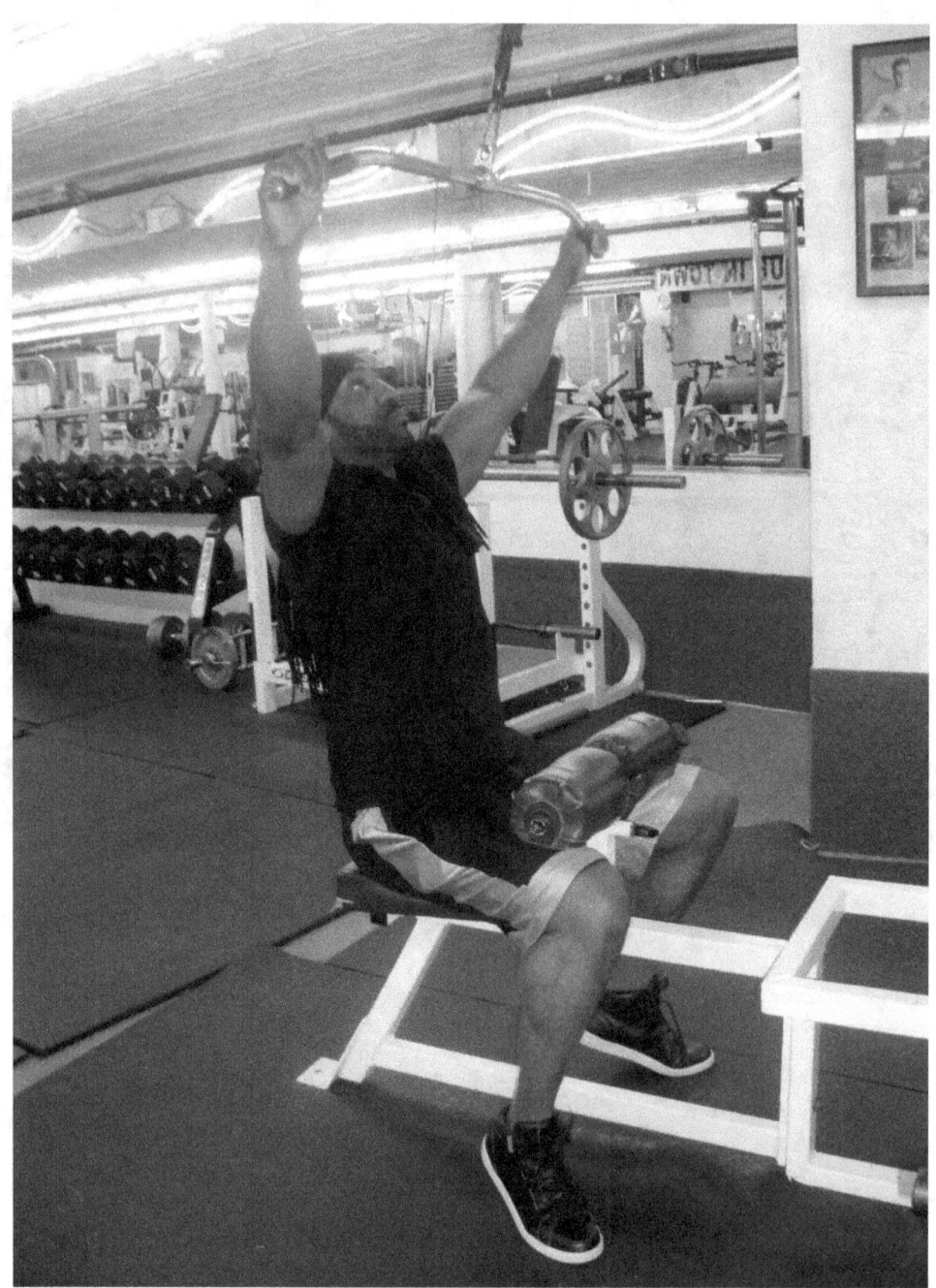

Lateral pull down 1

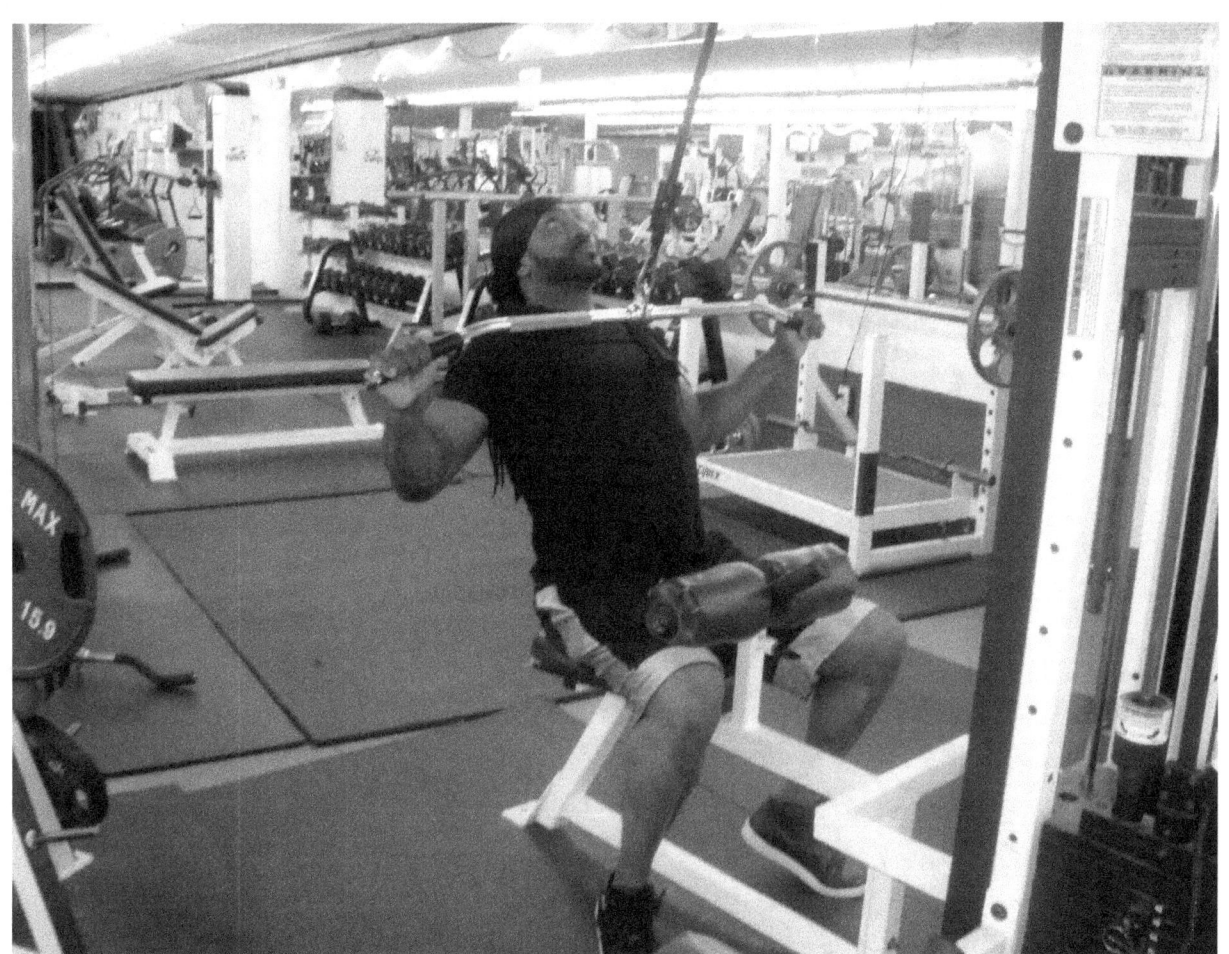

Lateral pull down 2

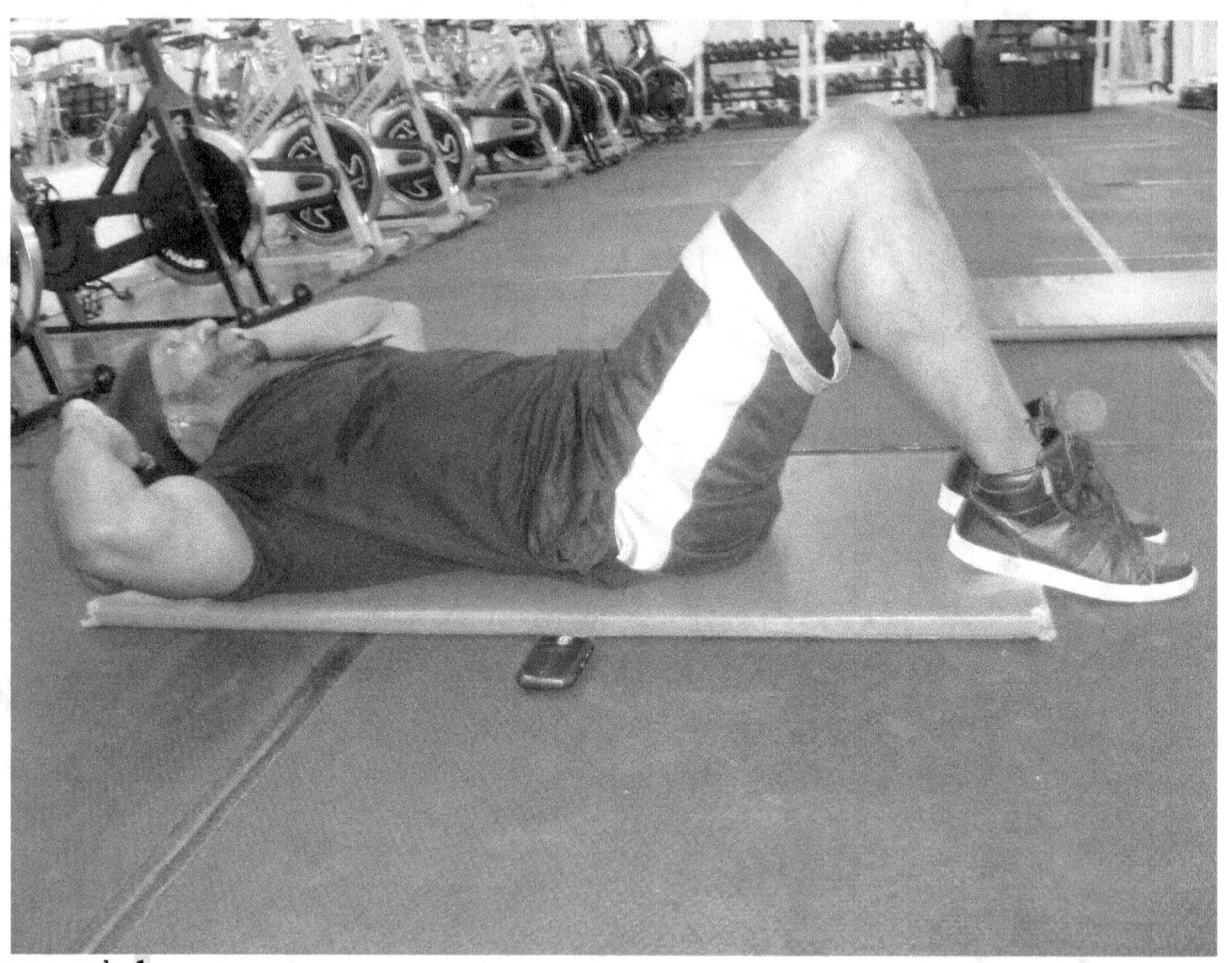

Laying crunch 1

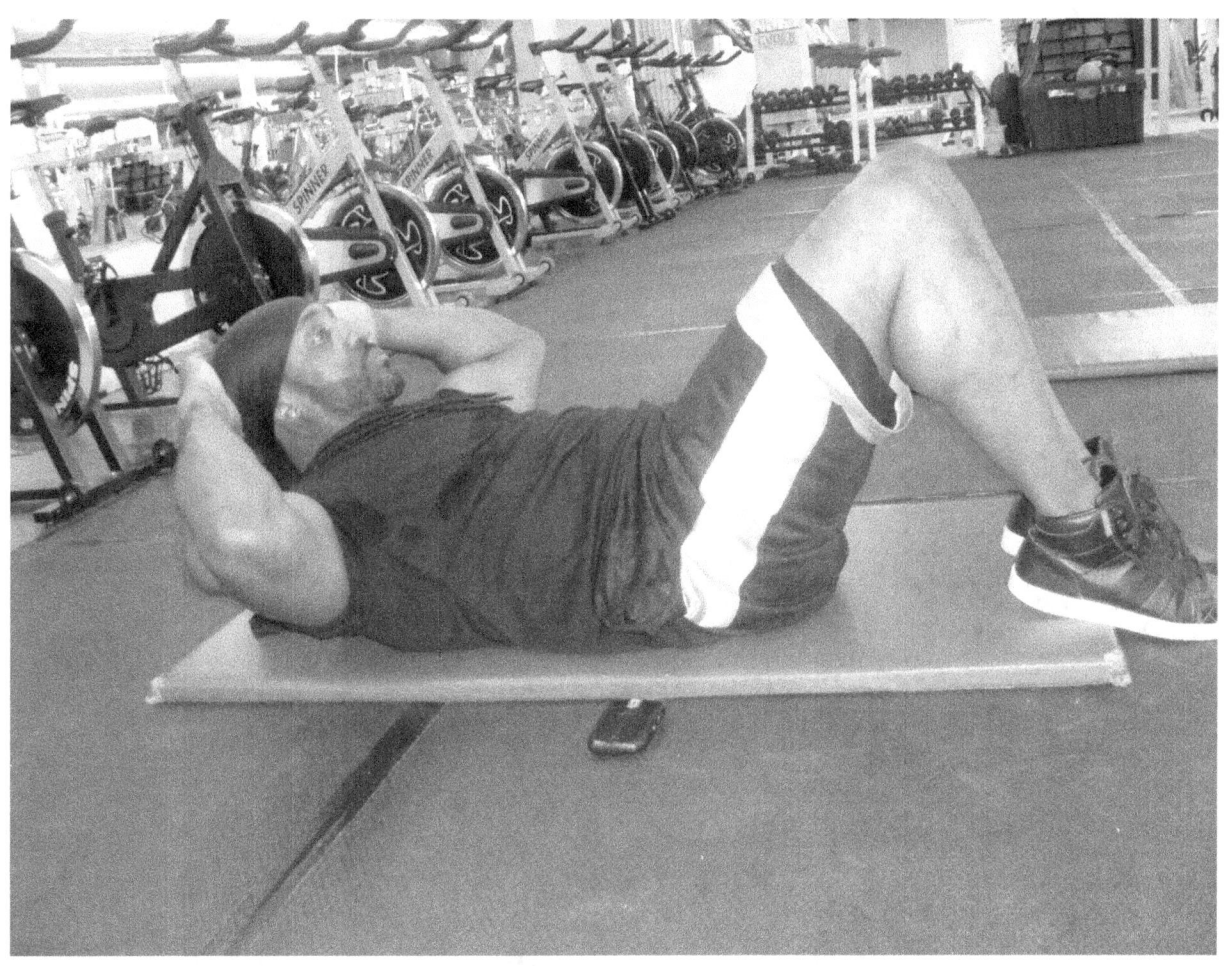

Laying crunch 2

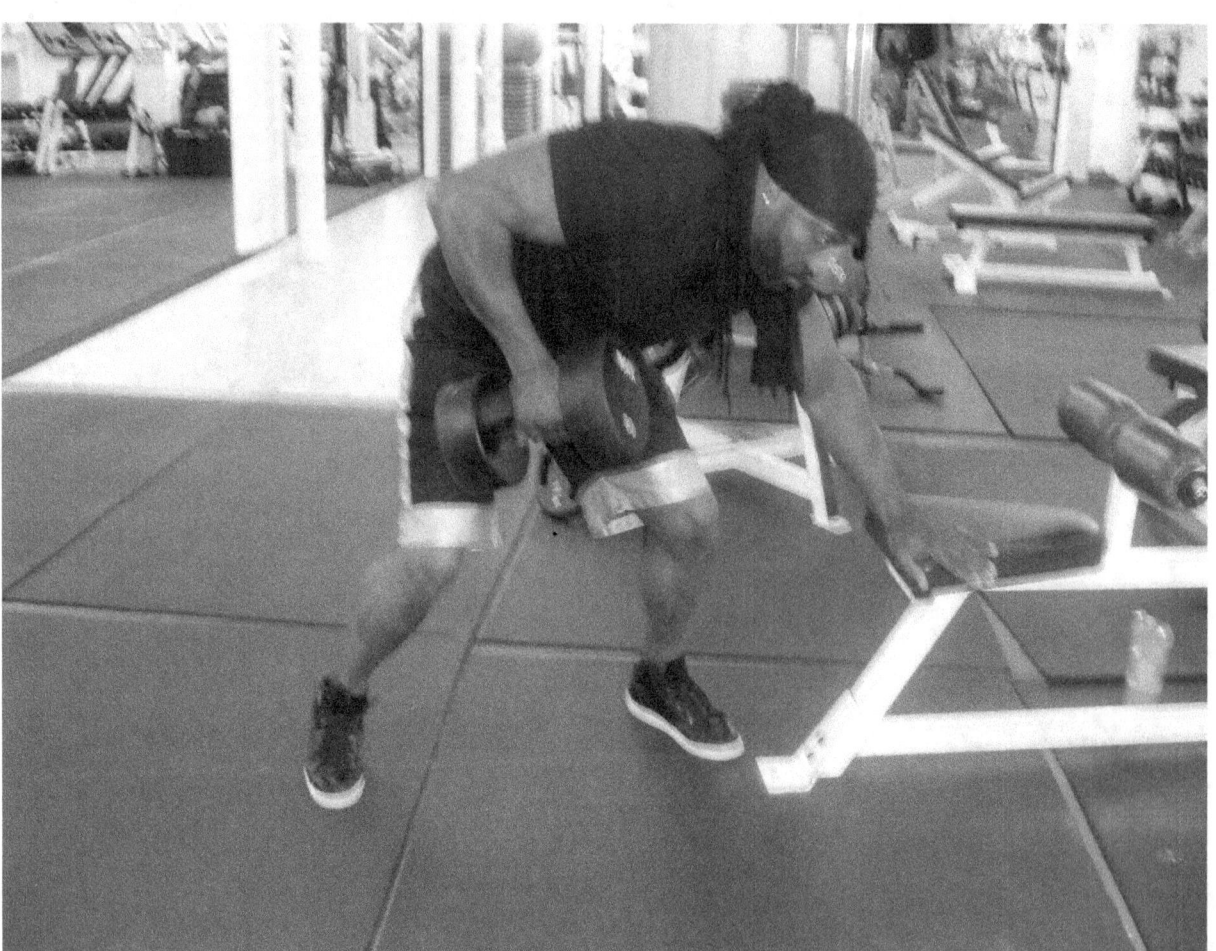

One-arm rows 1

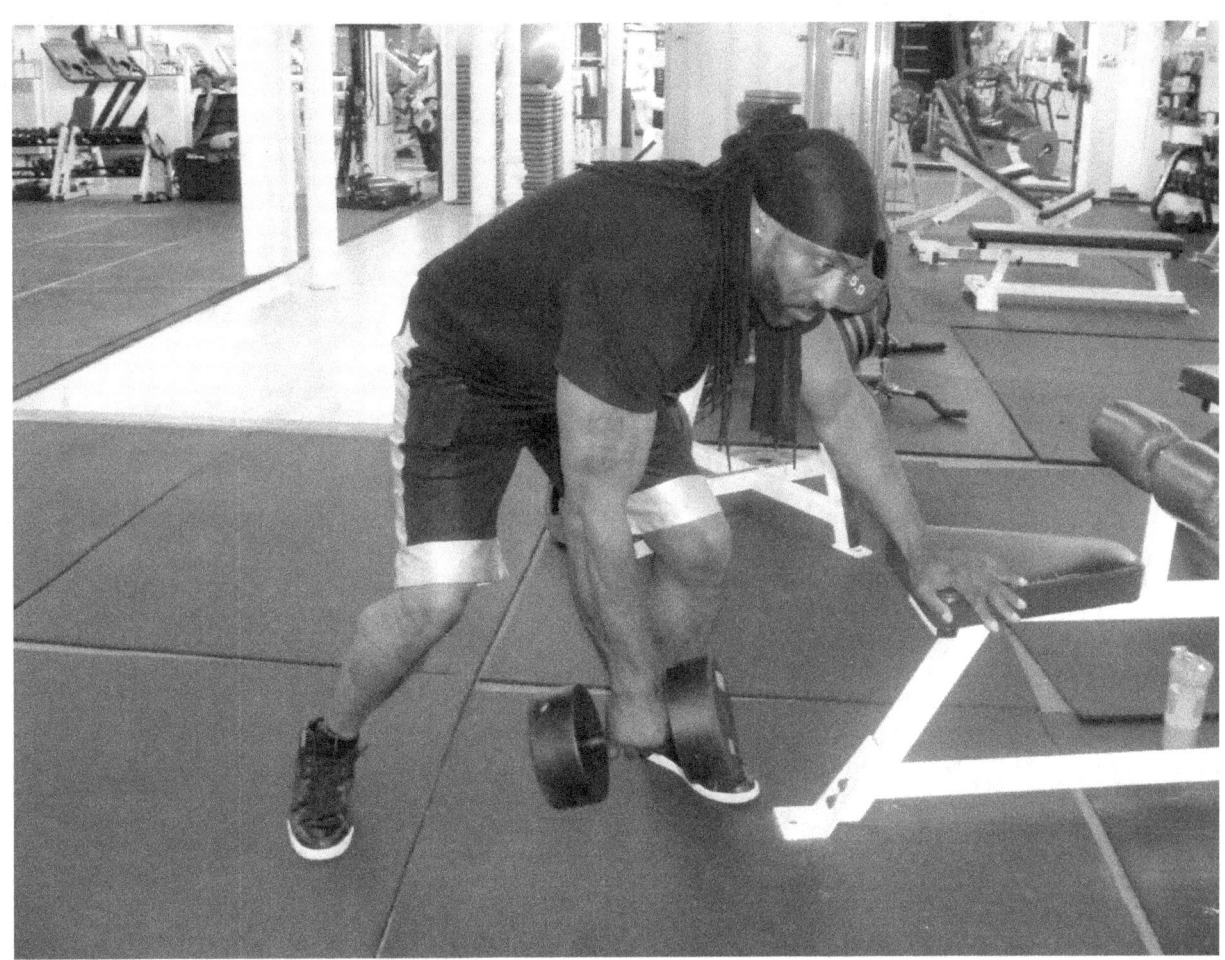

One-arm rows 2

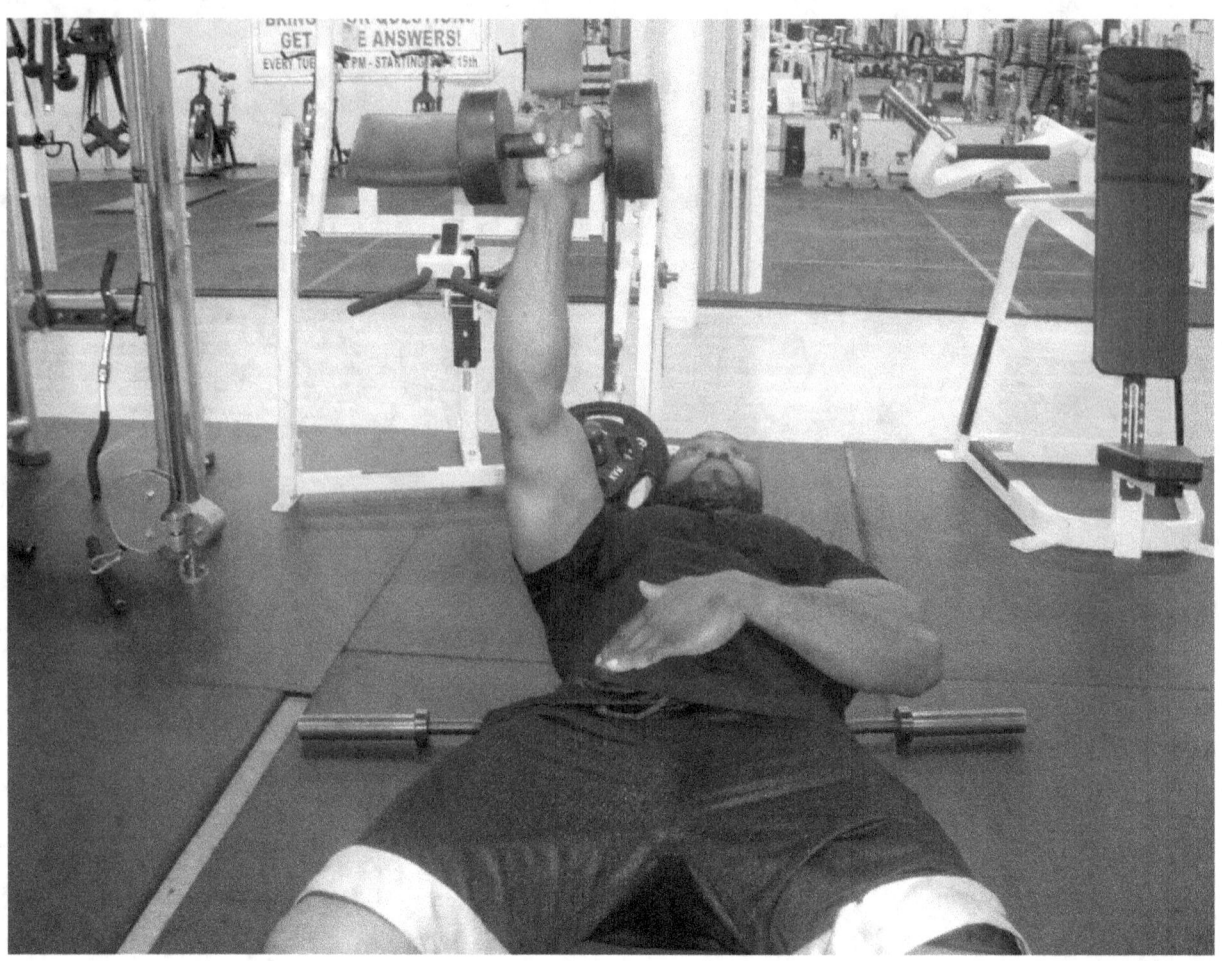

Dumbbell cross over 1

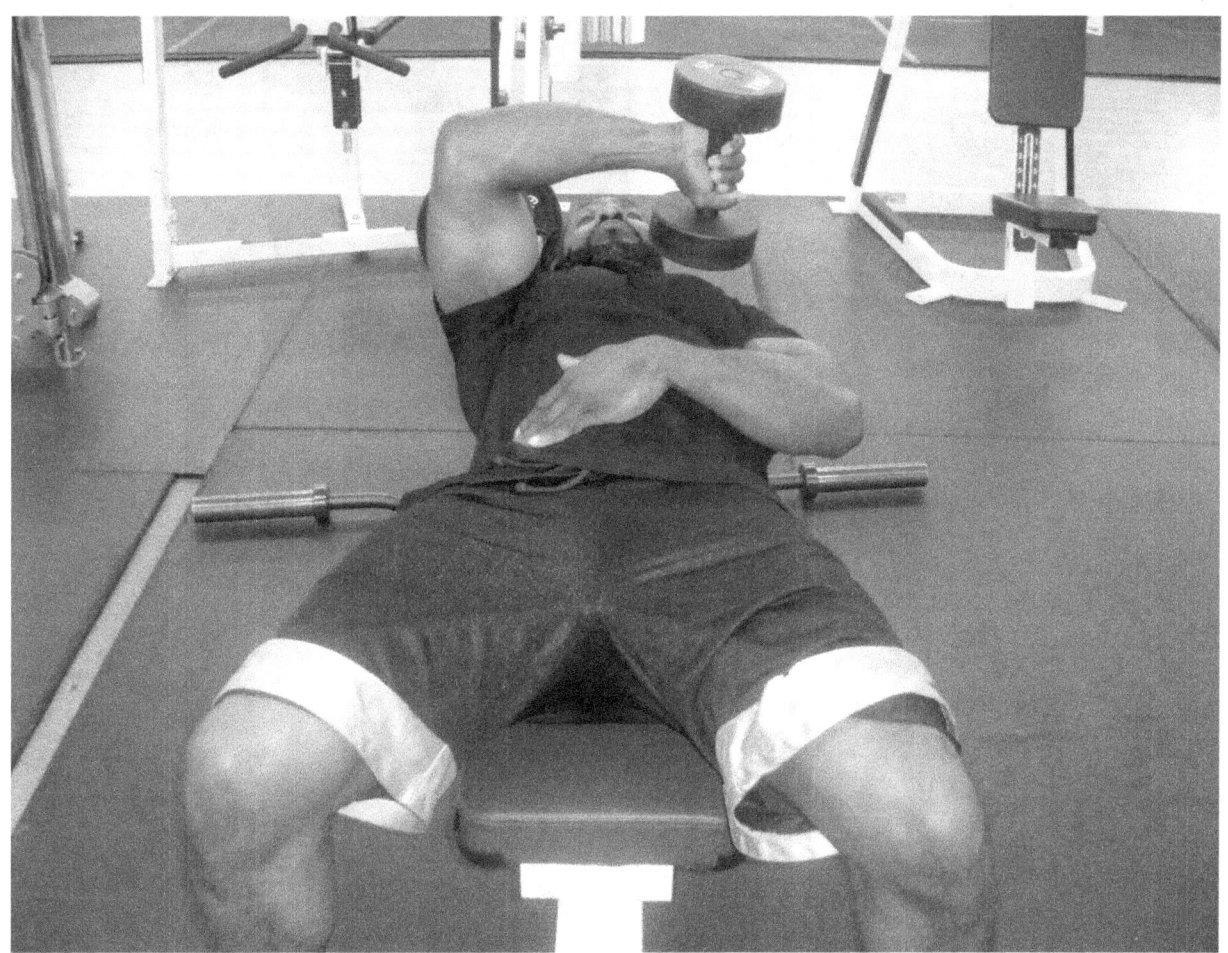

Dumbbell cross over 2

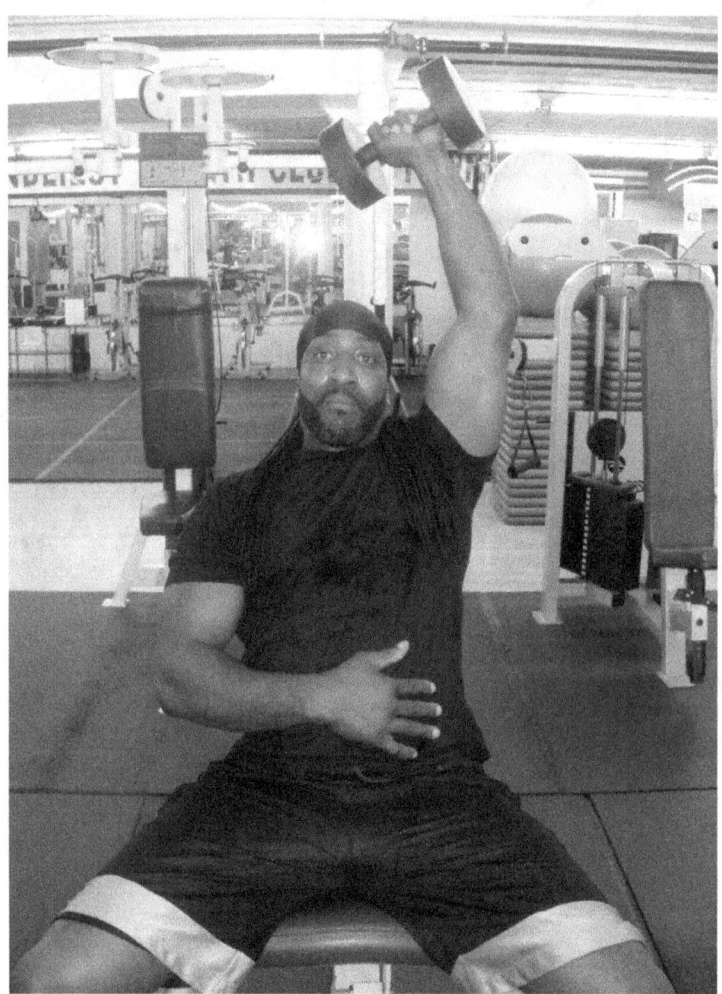

Seated tricep crossover 1

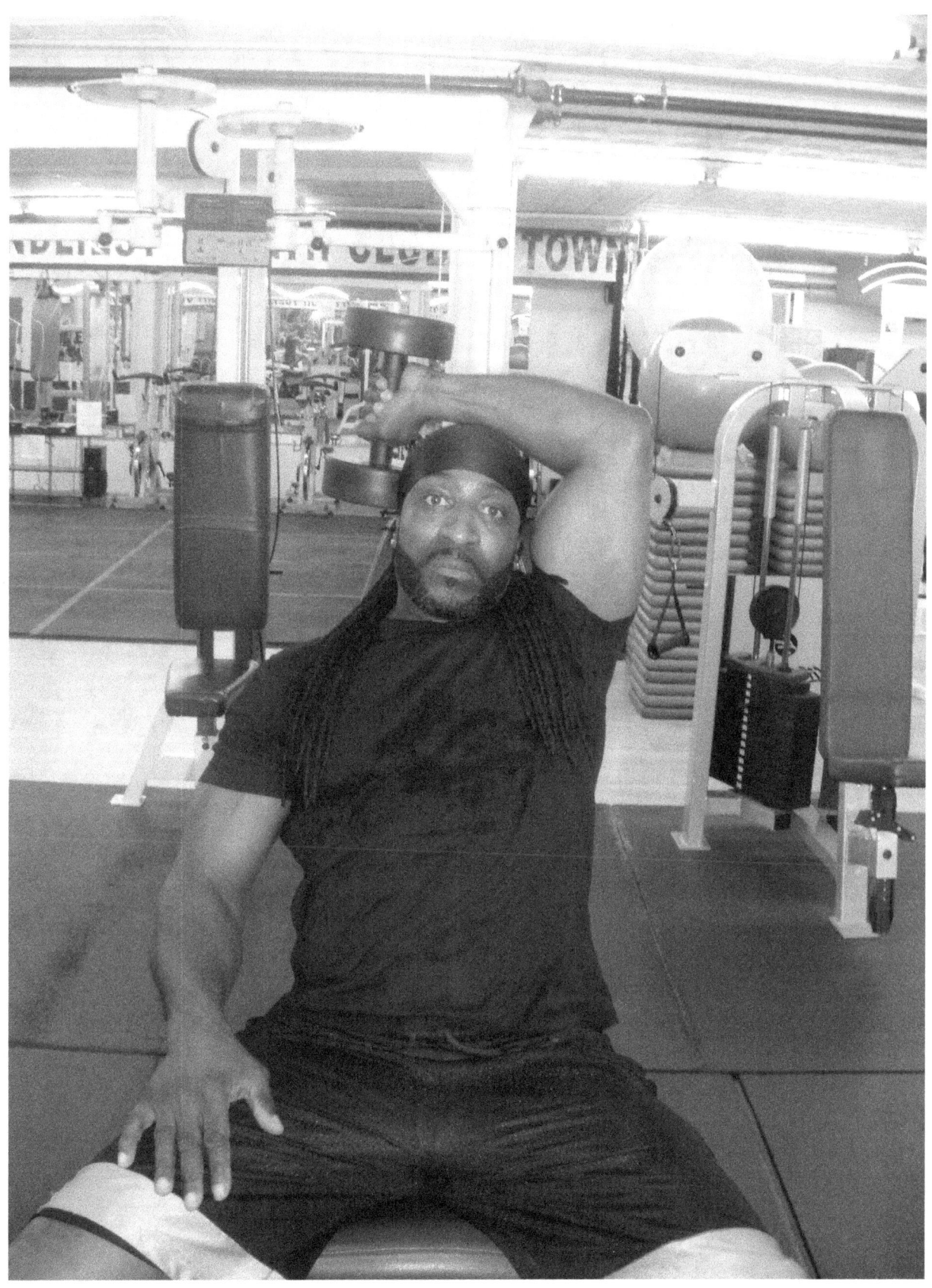

Seated tricep crossover 2

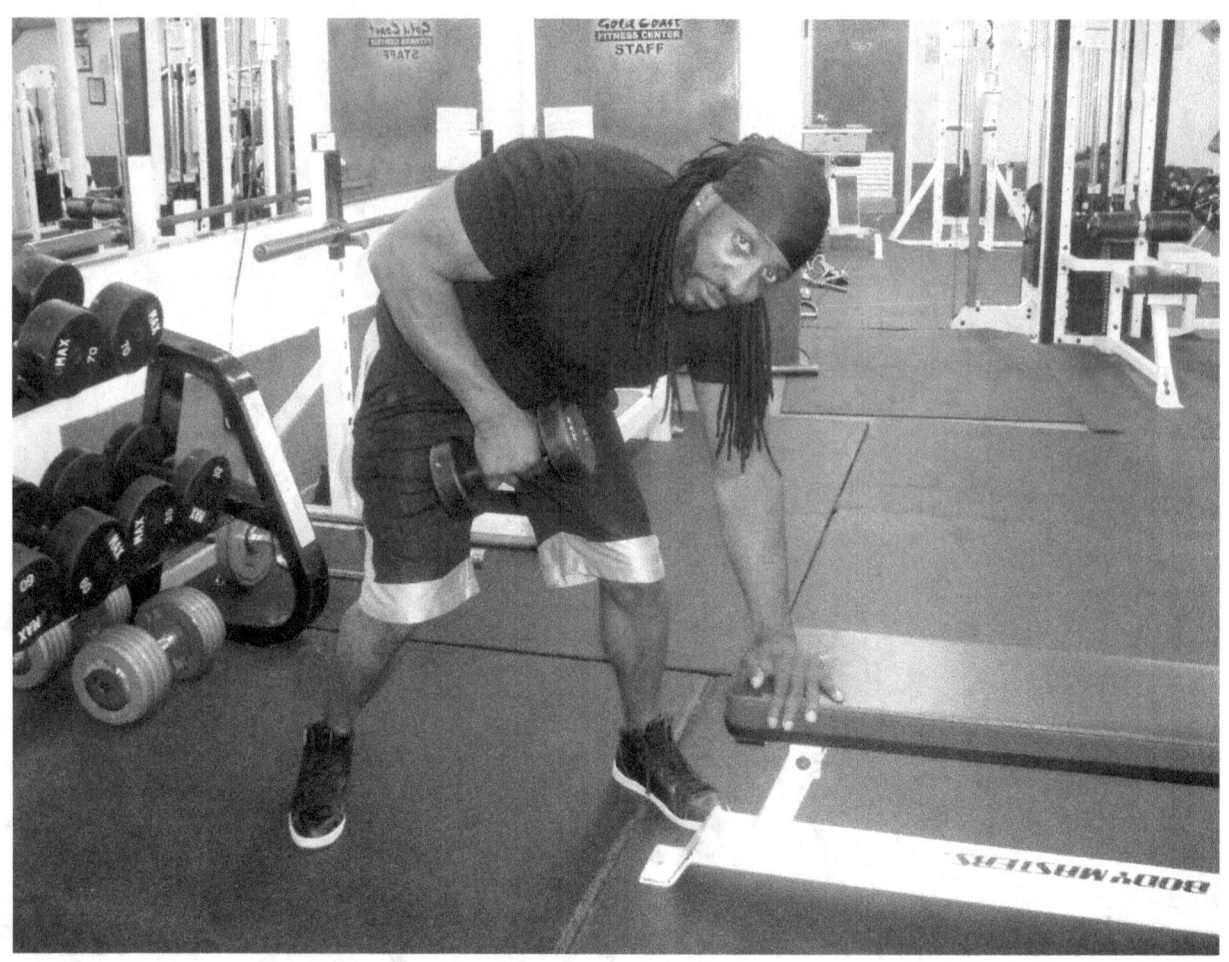

Tricep kick back 1

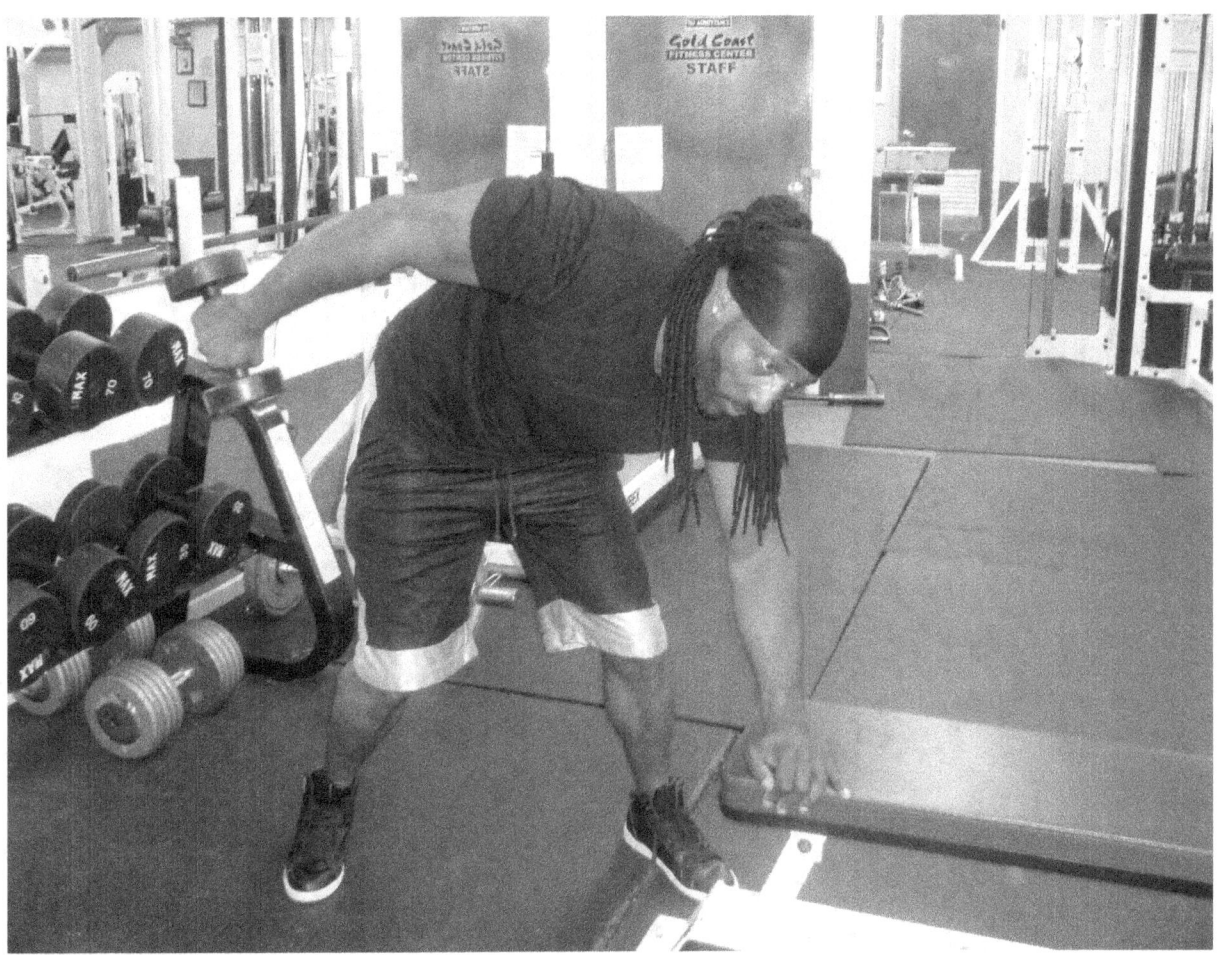

Tricep kick back 2

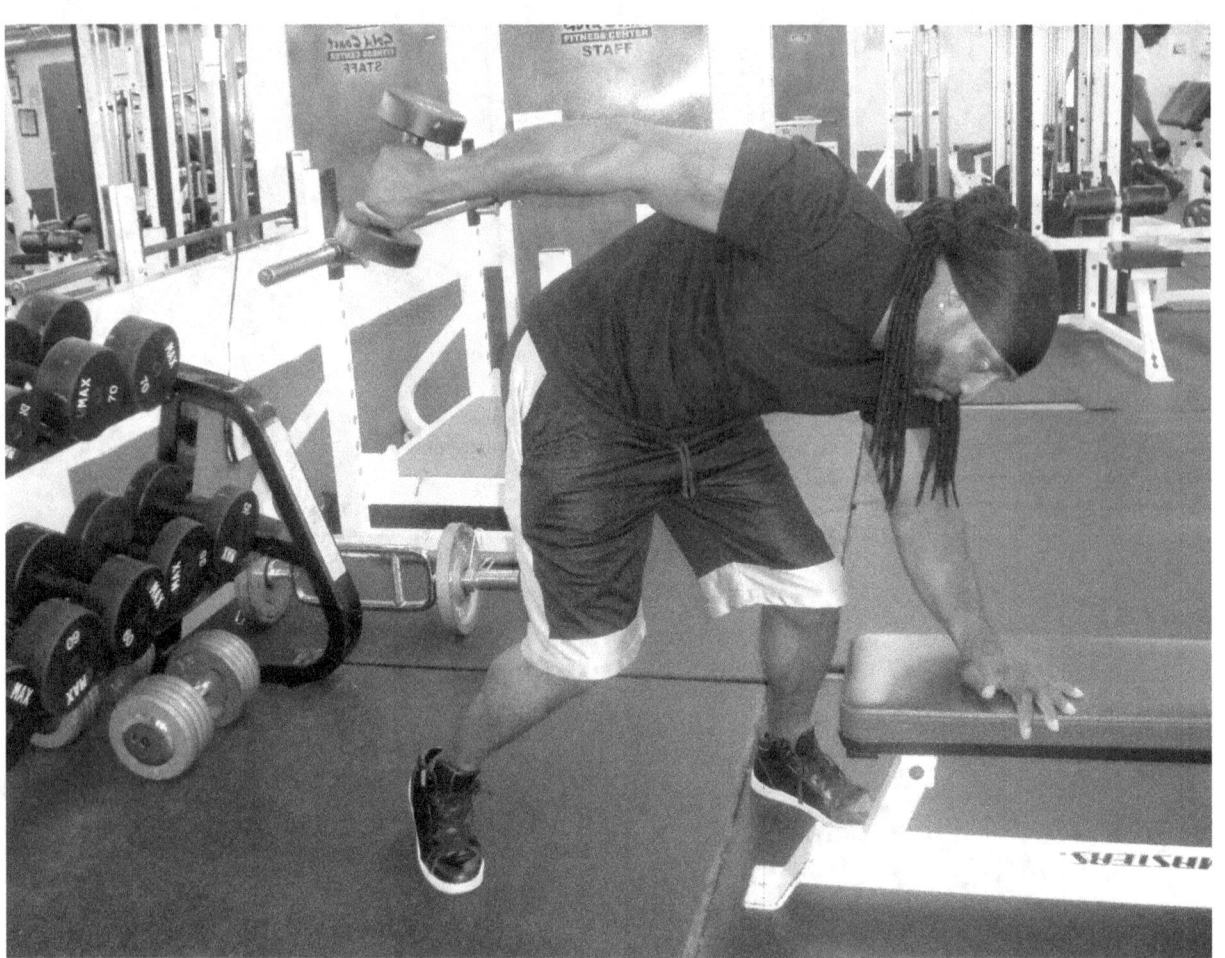

Tricep kick back 3

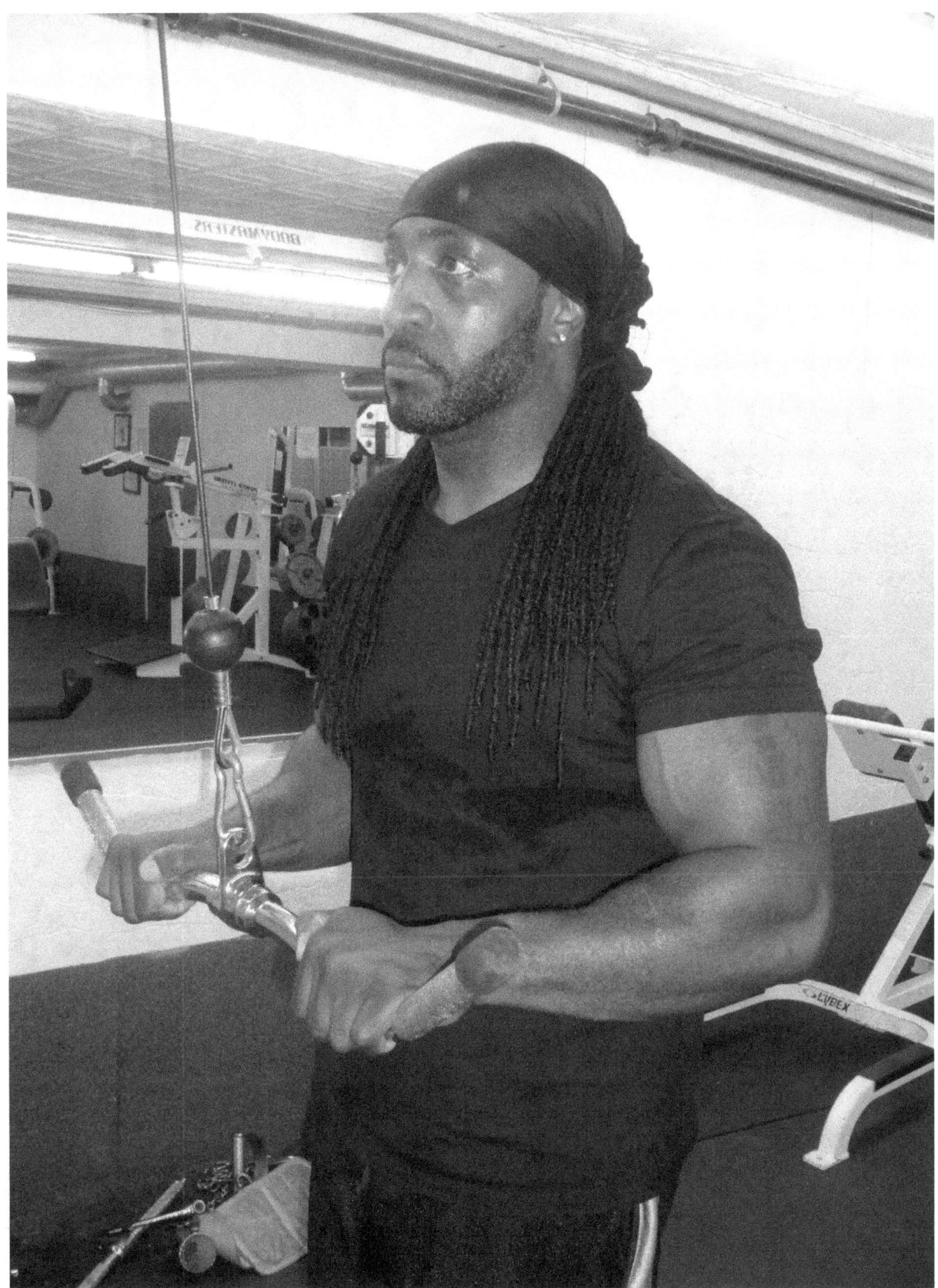

Tricep Press 1

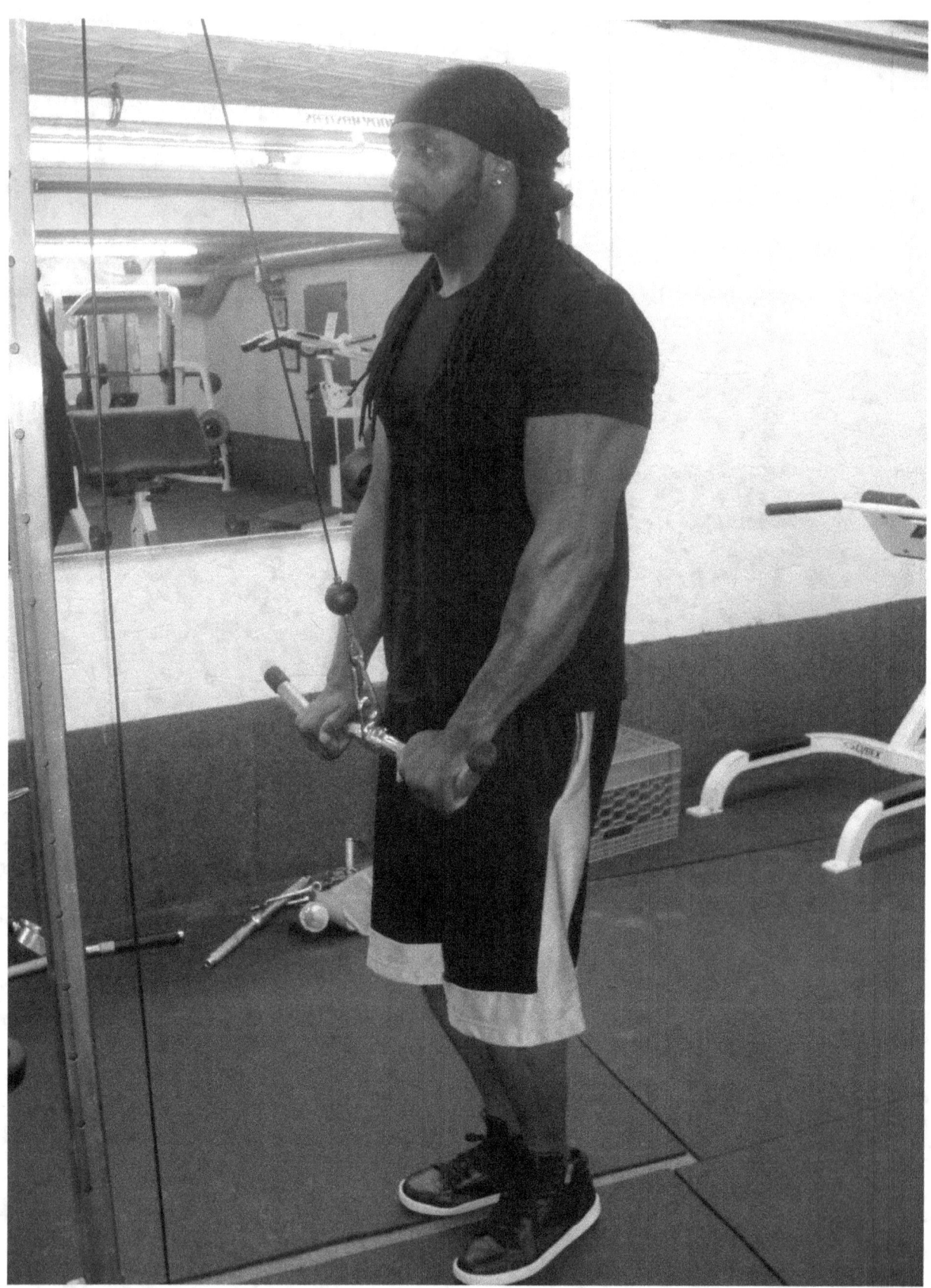

Tricep Press 2

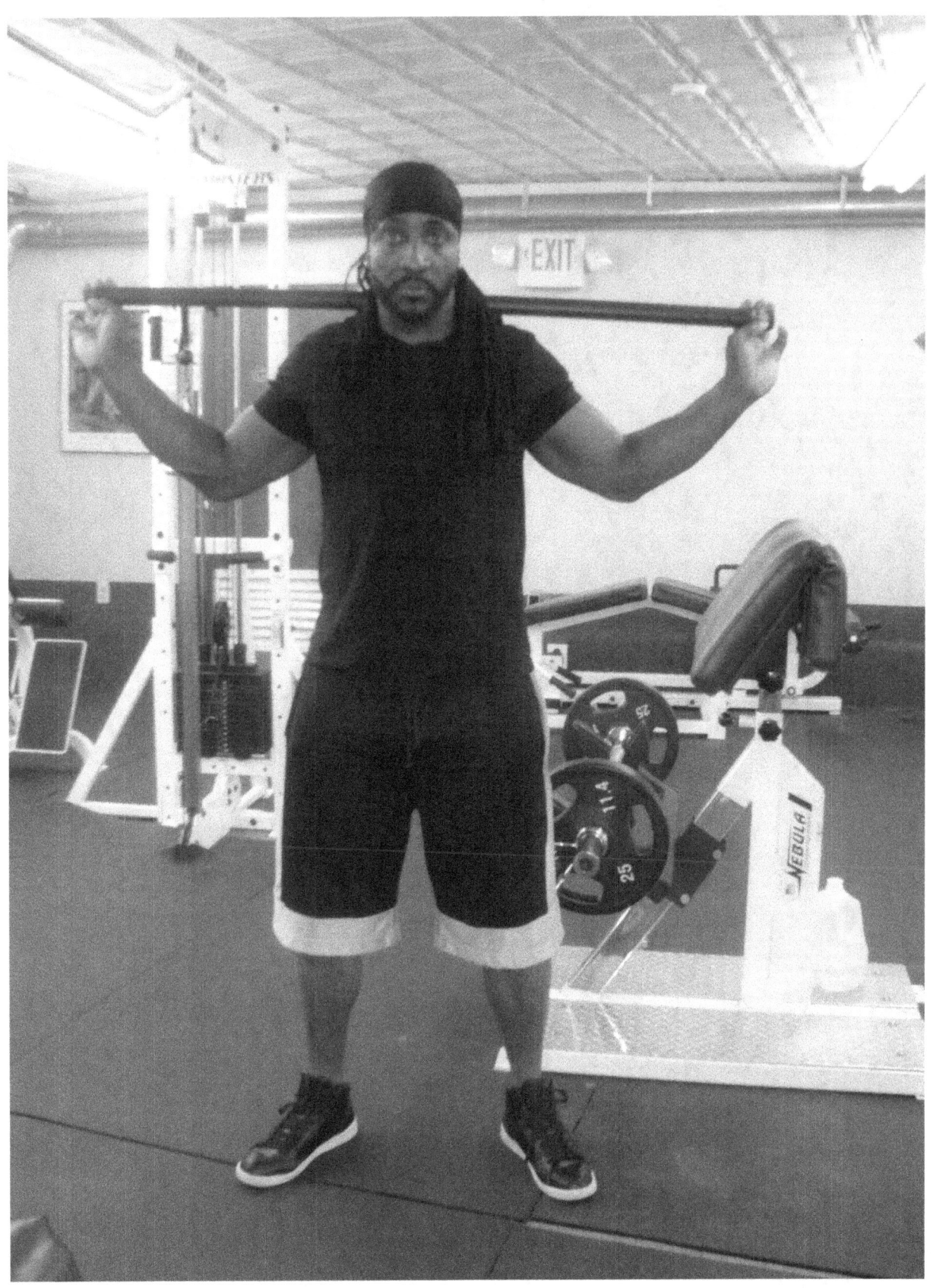

Standing Windmill